Augmentative Communication: Clinical Issues

Augmentative Communication: Clinical Issues

Susan M. Attermeier
Editor

The Haworth Press
New York • London

Augmentative Communication: Clinical Issues has also been published as *Physical & Occupational Therapy in Pediatrics*, Volume 7, Number 2, Summer 1987.

The Haworth Press, Inc., 12 West 32 Street, New York, NY 10001
EUROSPAN/Haworth, 3 Henrietta Street, London WC2E 8LU England

Library of Congress Cataloging-in-Publication Data

Augmentative communication.

"Has also been published as *Physical & occupational therapy in pediatrics*, volume 7, number 2, summer 1987"—T.p. verso.
Includes bibliographies.
1. Speech disorders in children—Patients—Rehabilitation. 2. Communication devices for the disabled. I. Attermeier, Susan M., 1942- . [DNLM: 1. Non-verbal Communication. 2. Self-Help Devices. 3. Speech Disorder—rehabilitation. W1 PH683P v.7 no.2 / WL340 A919]
RJ496.S7A84 1987 618.92'855 87-7557
ISBN 0-86656-657-0

Augmentative Communication: Clinical Issues

Physical & Occupational Therapy in Pediatrics
Volume, 7, Number 2

CONTENTS

Foreword

The inability to use speech as a primary means of communication due to central nervous system insult, progressive disease of the nervous system or any number of other physical and psychological reasons is devastating. Persons with severe expressive communication disorders endure severe penalties educationally, socially, vocationally and personally.

Ricky Creech has spent all of his life without the use of natural speech. His statement, using a speech synthesizer, relative to this issue is very powerful:

> I know of no other handicap as great or having as great an effect on a person's psychological and sociological development as being unable to speak . . . The person who can't speak is a person who is ignored, and a person who is ignored is a person who is stunted in his development . . . For 24 years my thoughts and ideas were held prisoner in a cell which was my body and I was isolated from all others . . . So does an Agency (person) have the right to deny another person the right of (speech) communication?

For many years parents, speech/language pathologists, teachers, psychologists, occupational therapists, physical therapists, social workers and other habilitation/rehabilitation specialists, have been concerned about finding appropriate augmentative/alternative communication systems for persons whose physical and neurological disabilities prevent them from using speech as their primary means of communication and interaction.

Creech puts the question of the right to have augmentative/alternative communication aids and techniques available quite directly. The impact of this question is particularly pertinent in a time when our knowledge of methods, aids, and techniques for providing augmentative/alternative means for communication has increased so greatly. For example, technology has advanced to the stage where even our automobiles, refrigerators, calculators and a variety of other household objects give commands to us using synthetic speech. Synthetic speech output is also available for the handicapped in the form of assistive communication devices. In addition to speech synthesis, sign language, gesture codes, microcomputers

---

David E. Yoder, PhD, is Chair, Department of Medical Allied Health Professions, Medical School Wing E 222 H, University of North Carolina at Chapel Hill, Chapel Hill, NC 27514.

and non-automated devices are available as communication systems. It is therefore the responsibility of the interdisciplinary team of specialists "fitting" a person with an assistive device to explore the complete array of augmentative communication systems available for use. Since communication is of such a high priority in our society today, it becomes extremely critical for us to look at the ways in which both natural speech and augmentative/alternative communication techniques and aids can become a functional output system for the severe speech impaired person.

Most all of the augmentative/alternative systems available for use by severe speech impaired persons require that the user have certain cognitive and motor skills. In some cases these requisite skills can be taught, but in other situations that is not possible. In other words, the cognitive and motor abilities of some persons may make augmentative/alternative systems as they are developed today inappropriate for them. For that reason we need to ask some basic questions of each individual whom we may consider a candidate for an augmentative/alternative communication system:

1. Will an augmentative communication system increase functional communication? (e.g., ease interaction and broaden social contacts)
2. Will an augmentative communication system facilitate interaction with persons in an educational, social, and vocational environment? (e.g., speech output and hard written materials)
3. Will an augmentative system provide for an increased level of independence? (e.g., answering phones; calling for help)
4. Will an augmentative system provide for learning of new communication skills? (e.g., language and syntax)
5. Will the augmentative system provide for a "personalized" vocabulary and means of unique expression?
6. Will the augmentative system provide for a less restrictive means of interaction than no formal system? (e.g., the closed interaction of signing versus the open system of speech output)

There is no perfect augmentative/alternative communication system. And there is no "perfect" set of materials to instruct those of us working with severe communicatively handicapped persons, on how to fit communication aids and techniques. The material presented in this volume is assembled by an interdisciplinary team, which has accumulated its base knowledge and information from experience with nonspeaking clients and their families. It is shared with the notion that individuals in need of augmentative/alternative systems will benefit from our shared knowledge and best data. Any augmentative/alternative system is only as good as the use to which it is put, and so it is the responsibility not only of the user, but also persons in the users' environment to adapt to the limitations of the system (e.g., reduced intelligibility of synthetic speech, slow information exchange, telegraphic sentences and poor written syntax). But augmentative/alternative communication allows for a personal interaction and also opens the door to communication for persons with severe expressive communication problems so they, like the rest of us, can eventually

> . . . talk of many things; of shoes—and ships—and sealing wax—of cabbages—and kings—and why the sea is boiling hot—and whether pigs have wings.
>
> (Lewis Carroll, *Through the Looking Glass*)

David E. Yoder

COMMENTS FROM THE GUEST EDITOR

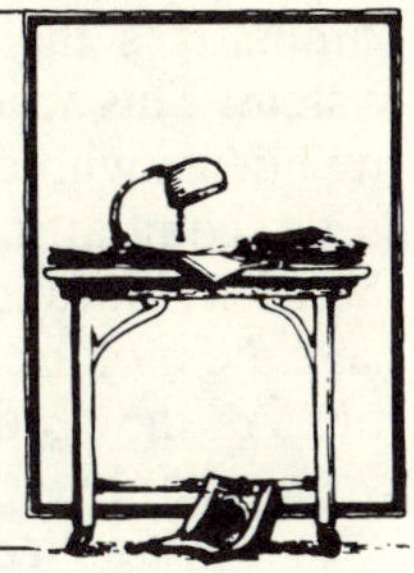

This issue of *Physical and Occupational Therapy in Pediatrics* is devoted to an area which is rapidly gaining recognition in all areas of rehabilitation – the field of Augmentative Communication. Provision of communication systems for non-speaking individuals is a fascinating and complex process which requires interdisciplinary cooperation. The authors have worked together for several years, primarily with young children, but also with adolescents and adults. Their intent is not only to inform clinicians as to the processes involved, but also to assist them in incorporating the concepts into their practice even if they are not members of a formal team.

In the United States, the American Speech-Language-Hearing Association (ASHA) is providing the primary leadership in augmentative communication, though clinicians in several different disciplines are involved in the effort. The purpose of this volume is not to restate or even attempt to summarize the work of ASHA, nor to discuss the array of technology available. Advances in technology are being made rapidly, and any information presented here would be obsolete by the time of publication; the equipment vendors listed in Appendix II will be an ongoing source of up-to-date information. The intention here is rather to supplement those sources by addressing a number of issues pertinent to the assessment and training of augmented communicators. Some of these issues have been previously addressed in the literature and are presented here in compact form. Other issues have not been previously addressed in comprehensive fashion, and the authors are basing their comments primarily on clinical experience.

In the first article, the guest editor describes the history and operating principles of augmentative communication. She also describes the structure and function of an evaluation team, and offers a series of suggestions for therapists involved in early intervention with handicapped infants and young children.

Nancy Johnson-Martin, a psychologist with many years of experience, summarizes the prerequisites for implementation of a communication system. This article will be of interest to anyone working with non-speaking clients who do not yet have a method of communication. Dr. Martin, in a second article with Pamela Wolters and Shelley Stowers, addresses the tricky question of assessing cognitive function in clients who do not have the motoric capability to take intelligence tests in standardized fashion. As the reader will note from the bibliography, few authors have written on this topic which presents constant problems to psychologists.

Jane Mac Neela, LPT, then presents a comprehensive review of the literature on positioning for handicapped clients in general as well as outlining the particular situations which must be accommodated if a communication system is to be compatible with the positioning devices. She has also reviewed and critiqued the rather sparse literature on positioning with augmented communication and points out a number of areas in which research is needed.

Shelley Stowers, OTR, and Mary Ruth Altheide, OTR, discuss the problem of finding a match between the motor capabilities of the client and the motor demands of various aided and unaided communication systems. This article will be extremely valuable to those assessing motor function, since it goes into considerable detail on the assessment process as well as providing further reference sources.

Patricia Porter, CCC-SP, presents methods for selecting an initial vocabulary, including a series of diagrams which demonstrate this process. In a second article she discusses a topic critical to the success of any communication system—that of communication versus language training.

Mary Ruth Altheide and Jean Livermore, MSW, offer comments on the need for, and methods for promoting the involvement of the family in the development of a communication system. They also discuss the very practical issue of assisting in obtaining funding.

Carolyn Eddins, MA, presents an extensive review of the literature on methods of interacting with augmented communicators, concluding her article with a series of interviews with system users and clinicians.

For those interested in further pursuing the topic of augmentative communication, several good sources of information are available, and are listed in Appendix II. Of these, ASHA should be considered the primary source for information on current theory, location of evaluation centers, and location of university programs where training for personnel is available. Information clearinghouses, publications, and a selection of equipment vendors are also listed.

Susan M. Attermeier
Guest Editor

Augmentative Communication: An Interdisciplinary Challenge

Susan M. Attermeier

SUMMARY. Provision of alternatives to speech for nonspeaking persons is a relatively new phenomenon, especially in the United States. Since the passage of PL 94-142, augmentative communication techniques have been seen as necessary, and are gaining widespread attention. The American Speech-Language-Hearing Association (ASHA) is taking the major leadership role in developing the theory and practice of augmentative communication. In the clinic, however, an interdisciplinary approach is critical. Physical and occupational therapists have important roles on these teams, as well as unique opportunities to prepare very young children for possible use of augmentative communication.

INTRODUCTION

Communication is a fundamental human activity. We communicate through movement – facial expression, gesture, laughing and crying. Speech, which develops over the first several years of life, is a singularly human and very rich form of communication, but is unavailable to many members of our society for a variety of reasons including congenital neurological disorders, progressive diseases and sensory deficits. When these individuals come into contact with members of the helping professions they present problems which cross disciplinary lines, and which demand solutions involving interdisciplinary cooperation. In response to this demand, the concept of the Augmentative Communication Team has been gaining momentum in recent years. At this point in time, fully functioning teams are scarce, since they require the services of a variety of professionals and are very labor intensive, therefore very costly. The benefits to non-speakers and their families, however, are enormous.

HISTORY OF AUGMENTATIVE COMMUNICATION

Prior to about the 1970s, little attention was paid to providing alternatives for speech. Porter[1] described two basic reasons for this. First, the

Susan M. Attermeier, MA, LPT, Clinical Center for the Study of Development and Learning, CDLBSRC, 220-H, University of North Carolina, Chapel Hill, NC 27514.

generally accepted theory was that language emerged from the shaping of early babbling into words, and later into sentences. Without the prerequisite "raw material" in the form of vocal output, the development of meaningful speech (i.e., language) was deemed unfeasible.[2-4] Second, there was a strongly held belief among language clinicians that provision of an alternative to speech would make a child "lazy" and would discourage the further development of speech. Intensive speech therapy was, therefore, the only acceptable mode of treatment for non-speakers.

These beliefs persisted until, in the late 1960s, they were refuted by research evidence. Speech came then to be seen as an accessory to language rather than a critical component.[4,5] Furthermore, the implementation of augments to speech was found in many cases to encourage speech; in no case did it diminish speech.[6-8]

As described by Yoder and Vanderheiden,[9] augmentative communication as we know it today can trace its evolution to developments in three separate areas which have converged in the last fifteen to twenty years. The first of these was the development, in a number of countries, of early language and communication boards, with the first comprehensive descriptions appearing in the literature in the 1950s.

The second area consisted of the development of sign and gesture systems for the hearing impaired, which were then utilized with motorimpaired and autistic populations. From these systems, other modified sign and gesture systems were devised for motor impaired individuals. The third area, developed primarily in Europe, consisted of systems for typing and environmental control for vocal motor-impaired individuals; this laid the groundwork for the sophisticated interfacing systems in use today, and was elaborated upon by Canadian workers before being imported to the United States.

In this country, the passage of Public Law 94-142 in 1975 provided the motivating force for implementing all these prior developments.[9] As handicapped children were placed in the public schools, the need for a variety of practical forms of communication became obvious. Thus, methods for indicating responses via pointing were supplemented by methods for writing and vocal output. The interdisciplinary team process, which is now almost taken for granted, arose in great part from the necessity to develop Individual Educational Programs for children with various combinations of cognitive, linguistic, motoric and emotional capabilities.

CURRENT STATUS OF CLINICAL PRACTICE IN AUGMENTATIVE COMMUNICATION

In comparison to other aspects of rehabilitation, the field of augmentative communication is still in its early stages of development. The challenges posed by efforts to develop communication systems for nonspeakers are enormous in terms of underlying theory, evaluation techniques, training techniques, and ongoing incorporation of technological advances. The primary leadership role in coordinating all these efforts has been assumed by the American Speech-Hearing-Language Association (ASHA), which in 1980 established an Ad Hoc Committee on Communication Processes and Nonspeaking Persons. The published position statement of this committee outlines the broad scope of its approach, as it presents the concept of the Communication System (Figure 1) consisting of techniques, symbol sets/systems, and communication/interaction behaviors.[10]

The reader will note that, at one time or another, the normal individual makes use of all the techniques listed, as well as several of the symbol sets and all of the communication behaviors. The augmented communicator, on the other hand, is restricted to certain options based on his or her particular configuration of handicaps. For any given individual, then, the provision of a communication system will involve:

1. careful assessment in terms of cognitive, linguistic, motoric and emotional capabilities, as well as the interaction of those factors;
2. assessment of the environment in which the individual operates, including the characteristics of the family, the physical set up of the home and school, and the social/community milieu;
3. selection of the optimal communication system;
4. training the individual in the technical aspects of the system as well as in strategies for interacting with other people; and
5. follow-up and ongoing assistance, including possible provision of adaptations to the system.[10]

The work of ASHA is ongoing and extensive. A nationwide two-year project, funded in part by the U.S. Department of Education, entitled "Leadership Training in Augmentative Communication" has been undertaken. The products of this project will provide a wealth of resources for all clinicians working with non-verbal clients, though the project is aimed specifically at school-age children. A detailed volume entitled *Augmentative Communication: An Introduction*, with an anticipated publication date of fall, 1986, will serve as a curriculum guide at the University level, as well as a resource for clinicians. As a companion to this volume, an annotated bibliography is being prepared, and will be available through ASHA. Finally, eleven model sites for evaluation and follow-up are being established.

Broadly stated, the goal of these activities is to develop guidelines and strategies, as well as prepare personnel, for providing non-speaking persons with appropriate and functional means of communication. For any

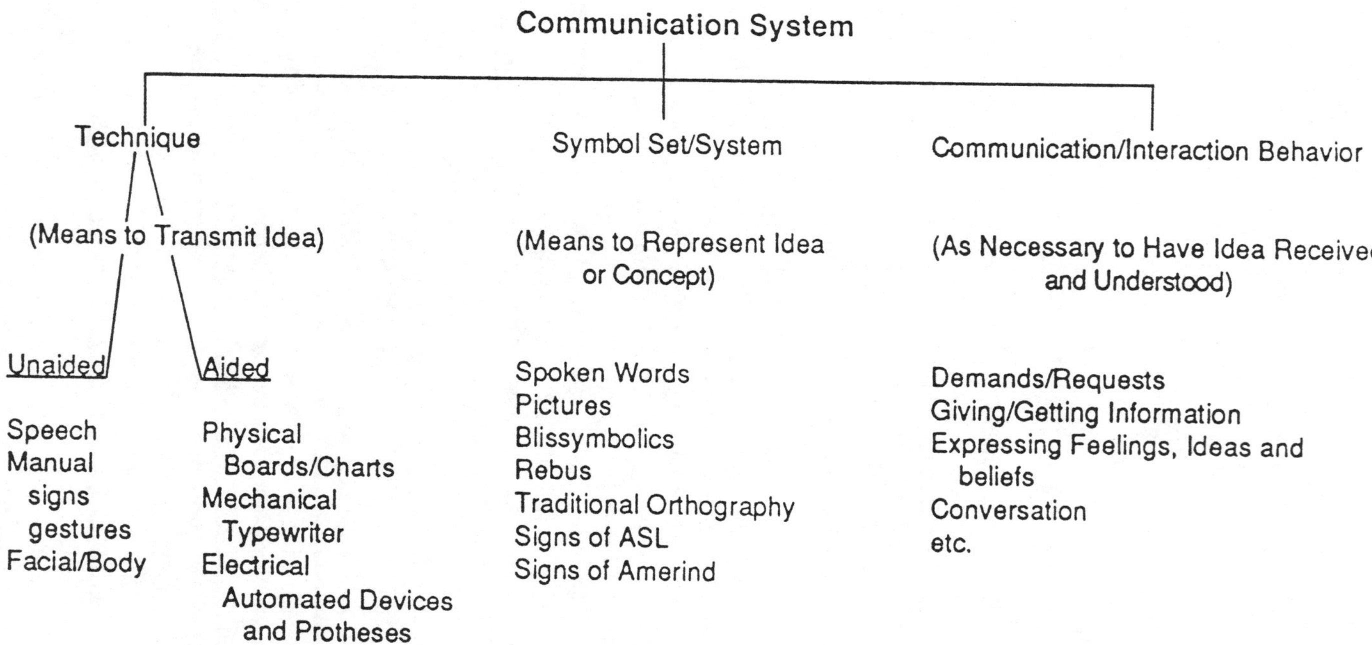

FIGURE 1. Components of a Communication System (reproduced with the permission of ASHA)

given individual, this will involve devising an array of options for use in different situations. This concept is referred to as the Multi-Technique-Strategy (MTS). Vanderheiden and Lloyd[11] have described the characteristics of an optimal MTS communication system, specifying that it should:

1. provide a full range of communication functions, including communication of basic needs, conversation, writing and messaging, and computer access;
2. be compatible with seating systems and all other positions, as well as mobility systems, environmental controls, and teaching devices;
3. not restrict communication partners, i.e., be usable with individuals or groups, familiar people or strangers;
4. not restrict communication environments or physical positions;
5. not restrict communication topic or scope;
6. be effective, providing maximum speed, a quick method for key messages, yes/no and basic needs communication at a distance, ability to interrupt and fight off interruptions, ability to avoid premature interpretation of a message, ability to overlay emphasis or emotion on a message, minimum fatigue, and special superefficient techniques for those close to the individual;
7. foster and allow growth in terms of topic, grammar, vocabulary and function;
8. be accepted and motivating to the user as well as the user's family, friends, and companions at school and work; and
9. be affordable in terms of purchase, maintenance, and need for an assistant.

CLINICAL CONSIDERATIONS

Team Function

Therapists, teachers, psychologists and social workers who work with children are frequently confronted with situations in which communication is an issue. The questions presented by parents are well-known: will she talk? when will she talk? how can we find a way to unlock the ideas in his head? Sorting out the answers to these questions is a process which requires not only skill on the part of the individual clinician, but also a commitment to the concept of interdisciplinary team function. The "fit" of a system to a particular child in his or her particular family/community environment requires much more expertise than any one person can have. Team members do not all have to be under one roof, though that is optimal. The critical factors are willingness to share roles and responsibilities, as well as defer to the expertise of other team members. Absolutely critical is the willingness to struggle through the difficult process of trial-and-error problem solving over a long period of time, for alas, there is no cookbook!

The make-up and roles of a team may vary somewhat, but the typical configuration is as follows:

> The *speech/language clinician* determines the status of language development and the extent to which speech is (or will be) a functional means of communication, selects the initial vocabulary to be used, selects an appropriate symbol system, and oversees the training of the individual and the family.
>
> The *psychologist* determines cognitive status, using formal standardized testing if possible and appropriate adaptations where necessary.
>
> The *physical therapist* carries out gross motor assessment with particular attention to seating arrangements and the extent to which they must be modified to facilitate use of a communication system.
>
> The *occupational therapist* carries out a detailed assessment of upper extremity function, looking for the most efficient mode of indication. (The physical and occupational therapists collaborate on assessing trunk and head function, particularly if eye/head movements are being considered as a response mode.)
>
> The *social worker* assesses family function in terms of strengths and stresses, and assists in locating funding sources.
>
> The *equipment vendor* provides equipment and devices on loan for trial during the evaluation, and orders the agreed upon pieces.
>
> The presence of a *biomedical* or *rehabilitation engineer*, should one be available, is extremely valuable for devising and constructing environmental control devices, and interfacing mobility and communication components (e.g., power wheelchair and electronic communication devices) with each other.

Depending on the particular client, these evaluations may be carried out singly or jointly. In any event, the process involves several steps. Preplanning, with information available on the client, family and school, and the specific questions to be addressed, is critical. At the time of preplanning, a community advocate should be identified. This should be someone who is familiar with the client's situation, and who is in a position to assist in local follow through. The community advocate attends the evaluation, and is considered to be a member of the team for that client. Following completion of the individual evaluations, the team meets as a group and comes to a consensus as to the next steps to be taken. After these decisions have been made, representatives of the team meet with the client and/or family to discuss the outcome of the day. This interpretation session may be difficult, particularly for a very young child, and may need to be extended over several sessions. If the parents are hearing a diagnosis of mental retardation for the first time they must be handled with great sensitivity, and can probably not be expected to absorb any more technical information at that session. In these situations, which are fairly common, the point needs to be made that the child can only communicate at his or her level of understanding, and that computers cannot put ideas into anyone's head. Even parents of non-retarded children need to understand that there is no technological "quick fix" and that the process of establishing communication systems is arduous and labor intensive.

Suggestions for Early Intervention Therapists

While the information in this volume will be of value to a broad range of clinicians and teachers, it can be particularly useful to physical and occupational therapists who work with infants and very young children. The non-speaking population consists to a very great extent of individuals with significant motor handicaps. When these are identified in infancy, it is the physical or occupational therapist whose services are most likely to be prescribed; speech therapists, psychologists, and teachers are frequently not called upon until the child is of school age. Therapists, therefore, are in a unique position to prepare a child to become an effective communicator, using the following guidelines.

1. Do everything possible to obtain reasonable head control. This is, of course, a cornerstone of treatment for all handicapped children, but head control takes on special importance for augmented communication. The child who can maintain an upright head, control head movements, and separate eye movements from neck movements will be a more efficient communicator.
2. Build choice-making into the program. As soon as possible, the infant should be presented with choices between toys or games, and should be given control over his or her activities in as many situations as possible. Parents can also be shown how to incorporate this idea into feeding routines and other activities of daily living (e.g., selecting clothing each day, choosing books to be read or television programs to watch). This will promote a sense of capability and independence in the child.
3. Develop a mode of indication. The optimal mode of indication is pointing with an isolated index finger; if this is not possible, the fisted hand can be used. These patterns do not have to be normal in

appearance; they only need to be functional, reasonably efficient, and reliable. If the upper extremities cannot be used, indication of choices with eye gaze, head turning or nodding should be taught.

4. Encourage family members to talk and read to the child even though the child is not talking. Because it is so easy to fall into the habit of not talking to a nonverbal child, family members should make a special point of including the child in conversations, as well as providing name labels for objects and helping the child learn that pictures can represent objects.

All of these suggestions can be easily incorporated into a therapeutic program. If the child does develop the ability to speak, nothing will have been lost; if not, the groundwork for augmentative communication will have been laid.

SUMMARY

The field of augmentative communication is a relatively new and rapidly evolving one. Although the primary leadership role is being assumed by ASHA, service to clients can only be carried out by means of an interdisciplinary team, using both individual expertise and group problem-solving. Physical and occupational therapists have indispensable roles on these teams, as well as a unique role in preparing very young children for use of augmented communication.

NOTES

1. Porter P: Aided augmentative communication for the non-verbal child: Necessity and efficacy. Unpublished manuscript, 1977.

2. Carroll JB: Language development in children, in Saporta S (ed): *Psycholinguistics: A Book of Readings*. New York, Holt Rinehart and Winston, 1961.

3. Mowrer OH: Speech development in the young child: 1. The autism theory of speech development and some clinical applications. *J Speech Hear Disord* 17:263-268, 1952.

4. Lenneberg EH: *Biological Foundations of Language*. New York, Wiley, 1967.

5. Fourcin AJ: Language development in the absence of expressive speech, in Lenneberg EH, Lenneberg E (eds): *Foundations of Language Development,* Vol. II. New York, Academic Press, 1975.

6. Archer L: Blissymbolics – A nonverbal communication system. *J Speech Hear Disord* 42:565-579, 1977.

7. McDonald E: Language foundations, in Vanderheiden G, Grilley K (eds): *Non-vocal Communication Techniques and Aids for the Severely Physically Handicapped*. Baltimore, University Park Press, 1977.

8. McNaughton S: Symbol communication program at OCCC, in Vanderheiden G, Grilley K (eds): *Non-vocal Communication Techniques and Aids for the Severely Physically Handicapped*. Baltimore, University Park Press, 1977.

9. Yoder D, Vanderheiden G: Overview, in Blackstone S, Bruskin D (eds): *Augmentative Com-*

munication: An Introduction. Rockville, MD, American Speech-Language-Hearing Association, working draft, in press.

10. Ad Hoc Committee on Communication Processes and Non-Speaking Persons: Position statement on nonspeech communication. *ASHA* 23:577-581, 1981.

11. Vanderheiden G, Lloyd L: Communication systems and their components, in Blackstone S, Bruskin D (eds): *Augmentative Communication: An Introduction.* Rockville, MD, American Speech-Language-Hearing Association, working draft, in press.

The Prerequisites to Augmentative Communication: Their Implications for Therapists and Early Interventionists

Nancy M. Johnson-Martin

SUMMARY. Most assessment and curriculum materials for handicapped children have been developed on the assumptions that speech will be the primary mode of communication and that the development of motor skills will parallel development in other areas. Neither of these assumptions is valid for the nonvocal, physically handicapped child. The therapist or interventionist, therefore, has few guidelines for preparing such a child to communicate. Based on a knowledge of the normal development of prelanguage communication skills, as well as experience with communication development in nonvocal children, the Augmentative Communication Team at the University of North Carolina at Chapel Hill developed a list of prerequisite skills for use of aided communication systems. These prerequisites not only serve as indicators of "readiness" for an augmentative communication system but can also serve as a guide for preparing a child to use an aided augmentative communication system. This paper describes each of the prerequisites in detail beginning with the child's demonstrating preferences and proceeding through his or her selecting one of four pictures to communicate a choice of objects or activities.

A major challenge to those working with nonvocal, motor-impaired children is to determine when and how to promote the development of communication skills. Most assessment tools and curricula for handicapped children contain lists of skills in the language or communication domain that operate on the twin assumptions that the child will use speech as his or her primary mode of communication and that he or she will be able to demonstrate an understanding of speech in the same way as do normally developing children (i.e., by following instructions involving motor acts or by speaking to answer questions). Operating on these assumptions tends not only to frustrate interventionists as they try to promote the development of many atypical children but also to limit our perspective on the nature of communication.

Nancy M. Johnson-Martin, PhD, Head, Psychology Section, Clinical Center for the Study of Development and Learning, University of North Carolina, Chapel Hill, NC 27514.

Communication entails much more than understanding and speaking words. It is a process by which people inform one another of their needs and opinions. It begins shortly after birth. Although words increase its power and complexity, it can take place in the absence of words or even sounds—through gestures, facial expressions, and directed eye gaze. This broad view of communication must be maintained in order to think clearly about assessment and intervention for children who are unable to make speech sounds and unable to follow directions involving motor acts.

Based on this perspective and a number of years of clinical experience with nonvocal, physically handicapped children, the Augmentative Communication Team at the University of North Carolina at Chapel Hill has evolved a model of communication development that provides a general basis for understanding the emergence of communication in all children. More importantly, however, it provides guidelines for promoting communication in children whose handicaps may preclude the use of speech as a primary means of communication. According to this model, communication is necessarily the product of an interactive process. A child will not attempt to communicate unless he has a need to do so and will not continue to try to communicate unless the attempts meet with some success. The need to communicate is based on having preferences or desires that can be met by another person. In order for a communicative interchange to be successful, each party in the interchange must have feedback from the other that indicates understanding. That is, the child must "signal" another person to indicate a need, the other person must be able to "read" the signal and respond, and the child must be able to let the other person know whether the response was appropriate. At the simplest level these communicative interchanges may involve the child's crying or wiggling to indicate discomfort, an adult's alleviating the discomfort, and the child's smiling or snuggling in response to the care. With success on this simple level the child develops a range of different signals and begins to use signals more selectively. Instead of signaling food preferences by open-mouthed acceptance or closed-mouth refusal she will signal choices between different foods by such methods as pointing, shaking the head, and making sounds. *Preferences* determine the first topics for communication. As the child progresses through the first year of life, interests are added to preferences as topics for communication and the number of communication episodes increases dramatically. Then, as the capacity for symbolic thinking (i.e., the recognition that specific sounds, words or pictures stand for objects or events) emerges near the end of the first year or beginning of the second, the child is able to communicate about *objects and events not immediately in the environment.* The child has added language to his communication repertoire, whether it is only an understanding of language or both an understanding and an ability to speak the language.

This model of communication development was the basis for the booklet, *Prerequisites to Augmentative Communication*[1] written by the Augmentative Communication Team to describe the characteristics or skills that are essential to a child's success in using a communication board at a symbolic level. The book was designed to be a guide to practitioners as they prepare children for use of an augmentative communication device. For the purposes of this chapter the booklet provides a good outline for expanding a discussion of the model described above and its implications for working with nonvocal children. According to the booklet, a child is prepared for an augmentative communication system after he or she (1) has demonstrable preferences, (2) is "reinforceable" by objects or events that can be represented by objects or pictures, (3) has at least one signal or mode of indication, (4) will use the signal to indicate a desire for an object or event, (5) will use the signal to indicate a choice between two objects or events, (6) will use the signal to indicate a choice between four objects or events, (7) will use the signal to indicate a choice between pictured objects or events and (8) will use the signal to indicate a choice among three or more pictured objects or events.[1(p3)] Each of these prerequisites will be discussed below.

The child must have preferences. As noted above, a person who has no preferences has no need to communicate. Regardless of how handicapped a child may be, establishing a list of preferences is critical. Preferences may be for one person over another, one position over another, or one food over another. Preferences may be determined by indications of attention or pleasure on the one hand, and by indications of withdrawal or displeasure on the other. A list of such preferences indicates possible topics for the beginning of communication.

The child must be reinforceable by objects or events that can be represented by objects or pictures. The term "reinforceable" means that the child changes her behavior as a result of the consequences of that behavior, i.e., she "learns." For example, if the child reaches out with her arms toward a parent and is picked up, she is likely to learn that reaching out is a way to communicate "I want to get up." If she increases the rate of reaching out to a parent after having been picked up, we can say that the child is reinforceable and that being picked up is a "reinforcer." Clearly, the ability to communicate is based on the ability to learn that different actions have different effects on the environment, especially that certain actions influence what other people do.

The normally developing child has many opportunities to experience reinforcing events in the environment. Through normal motor activity (e.g., kicking) he may activate a mobile or other toy, notice the effect and increase that motor activity. Through natural gestures (e.g., reaching toward a desired object) or particular sounds (e.g., cries, grunts, words) the child activates adults to do things for him. In contrast, the severely handicapped child has a very limited range of motor and vocal behaviors and, consequently, a limited number of opportunities to learn that he can control events in the environment. Many of these children become very passive and may appear to have neither an ability to learn nor a desire to communicate.

In such a situation intervention may need to focus on helping the child gain some control over the environment, whether or not such control is directly related to communication. The preferences identified in step 1 are likely to be reinforcers to the child and can, therefore, be paired with a particular child behavior in order to determine if the child can change her behavior on the basis of its consequences. For example, if a child has smiled or otherwise shown pleasure in hearing music, a switch may be mounted to the side of her head so that a slight turn of the head will make a tape recorder come on. If, over a period of time, the child turns her head in that direction much more frequently than before the switch controlled the music, we can say that the head turning has been reinforced by the music. This is a demonstration that the child is reinforceable.

One caution must be kept in mind, however, as one attempts to evaluate whether a child is reinforceable. One can *never* assume that any object or experience will be a reinforcer for a child even if it has appeared to be one of his preferences or has been demonstrated to be reinforcing to almost all other children. For example, a child may move his mouth toward banana pudding and turn his head away from spinach, clearly indicating a preference for pudding. The pudding, however, may not be a successful reinforcer for moving his hand toward a picture or for doing any activity other than eating. In order to determine whether the child is "reinforceable," one must experiment with many combinations of potential reinforcers and behaviors to be reinforced. Especially critical is that the behaviors to be reinforced be under the child's voluntary control. When working with very severely handicapped children, the careful pairing of reinforcers and behaviors may be the best way to determine which behaviors are under voluntary control as well as to determine how readily reinforceable a child is.

Note that the issue for this prerequisite is not only that the child be reinforceable, but that she be reinforceable by objects or events that can be represented by objects or pictures. This proviso is made because communication devices are based upon objects or pictures. The burden for satisfying this aspect of the prerequisite is more on the therapist than on the child. Almost anything can be represented by an object or picture; the task is choosing an object or picture that can be readily distinguished by the child and associated with the reinforceable object or event. For example, a parent's hand with two fingers outstretched, a clay model or a picture of a similar hand may stand for tickling; a piece of sandpaper or a picture of the sandbox may stand for going outside. The challenge is greater for a visually impaired child where shape and texture may need to be the salient features of objects, but with ingenuity the challenge can be met.

The child must have at least one signal or mode of indication. In order to communicate a person must have some consistent, observable method of indicating a response. Normally developing children have many forms of indication—a variety of gestures, movements toward objects or people, sounds, and directed eye gaze. In children with severe physical handicaps the number of reliable communication signals is greatly reduced. The simplest signals available for use in an augmentative communication system are pointing, reaching and looking. In evaluating the usefulness of a child's available behaviors as signals for communication, one must look at a variety of factors: is the behavior under voluntary control? Can the behavior be "read" (identified readily) by potential receivers of communication? Is the behavior reasonably efficient (how long does it take the child to act and how rapidly does he fatigue)? What is the physical range of the behavior? That is, if the child is pointing, to how many places can he point reliably, and what must the arrangement of those places be for efficient pointing? If he is using eye gaze, how far apart must stimuli be to allow a message receiver to be sure where the gaze is directed, and how many places can be used? These factors will determine the kind of communication system the child will be able to use as well as how readily he can progress through the steps toward using any augmentative communication system.

It is necessary for communication specialists to work closely with occupational and physical therapists to satisfy this prerequisite. These therapists will position the child and determine optimal modes of indication. Adequate positioning has been estimated to be more important than any other single factor in improving a child's ability to use a communication device.[2] Similarly, an evaluation of the efficiency and range of a child's potential signals in different positions will have a major impact both on the kind of device that can be used and on how effectively it will be used. These factors are discussed in more detail in the paper in this volume by Stowers and Altheide.

The child uses the signal to indicate a desire for an object or event. Once a reliable and readable signal has been identified and the physical range of the signal is understood, one must ascertain whether the child can use that signal to communicate a desire for an object or event. For example, if a mechanical toy is placed in front of her, will she look at it or point to it in order to get an adult to activate it? Likewise, if food is placed in front of her, will she use the signal to get the adult to begin feeding her? As noted above, some children may have learned to be so passive that they simply wait for something to happen without using a signal clearly within their capabilities. If this is true, one may need to "shape" a child to use a signal by physically guiding her to make the response and then immediately reinforcing the response with the object or event. Again, one may need to experiment with a variety of objects or events to be sure that the child is actually interested in those that are being presented. One must also be careful not to assume that the child is "too retarded" to master this step if it is not learned quickly. The older a child is and the longer history she has had of passively waiting for events to occur, the more difficulty she may have in learning that active participation is effective in changing the environment.

The child must use the signal to indicate a choice between two objects or events. Making choices is a major achievement both from the standpoint of cognitive and communicative development and from the standpoint of personal growth. Normally developing infants have many opportunities to make choices. When only a few months old they usually have opportunities to choose which of several toys to pick up. As they begin to move, they have some choice of where they are and what stimuli are available to them. They actively reject activities they do not like. In contrast, the handicapped child is often placed and left in one place for long periods, is helped to play with a toy of an adult's choice, and is generally regulated by adult preferences.

The major issues to be considered for this prerequisite are a child's ability to scan the choices so that he knows what the choices are, and the ability to use the signal to indicate a choice within a reasonable period of time. The best way to determine if the child is making a considered choice is to present him with a choice between a known preferred object (e.g., pudding) and a known nonpreferred object (e.g., spinach). The child must always be given whatever he has indicated is the choice. One cannot assume that it was the "wrong" choice unless the child communicates disappointment with what he receives. If disappointment is indicated, the choices may be offered again to see if a "better" choice is made. The decision that a choice is or is not "correct" must be made only on the basis of feedback from the child. *It must never be made on the basis of the adult's predictions about the child's preferences.* One may need to give the child many choices before one can determine that he is making careful and deliberate choices.

The child must use the signal to indicate a choice between four objects. The point of this prerequisite is the child's ability to scan up to four objects and make choices among them. Expanding beyond two choices is necessary if the child is to have a flexible communication system. Again, the only real measure of the "correctness" of the choices made by the child are her indications of pleasure or disappointment with what she receives as a result of the choice.

The child must use the signal to indicate a choice between two and then between three or more pictured objects or events. An augmentative communication device can be developed for a child who is able to choose between objects but not between pictures. The flexibility that comes from the use of pictures or other symbols is critical to the development of most complex systems, however. Thus, the last two prerequisites involve the child's moving from making choices between objects to making choices between pictures that stand for objects or events. The procedures for assessing whether the child has mastered these prerequisites are similar to those for choosing between objects. The child is presented with pictures and asked, "Which one do you want?" He is given the object or event represented by the picture chosen.

Note that in none of the prerequisites is any mention made of the child's receptive vocabulary. The child is not trained to "show me the pudding" nor to "show me the spinach" before he is asked to choose between them. During choice-making opportunities the objects are named for the child as they are placed before him but the question is always "Which one do you want?" Not identifying receptive vocabulary as a prerequisite to augmentative communication is a deliberate deletion. Very often interventionists attempt to prepare a child for augmentative communication by training him to look at (or point to) pictures or objects when they are named. In this manner the child's receptive vocabulary may be increased but the child's ability to communicate has not been improved and, in some cases, may have been further impaired by teaching him to follow instruction passively but to make no requests or statements. In some cases the child will learn to hate a "language board" because it stands for dull, repetitive training rather than for access to communication. Furthermore, we must attempt, in so far as possible, to teach communication to the handicapped child in the same way it is learned by the normally developing child. The normally developing child does not acquire her receptive vocabulary by drill but by having adults name and talk about things she is looking at, playing with or otherwise indicating an interest in; or by having adults call her attention to something and then name it, show how it works, or talk about it. If the handicapped child uses a signal to get an adult to do something for her or to make a choice, and if the adult then acts responsively and talks to the child about these activities and choices, the child will acquire receptive vocabulary in a way similar to that of the normally developing child. These more "natural" experiences give vocabulary much more personal meaning and communicative power.

IMPLICATIONS FOR EARLY INTERVENTIONISTS

Therapists and interventionists working with young, significantly handicapped infants often have no way of predicting the extent to which a given infant will become a vocal communicator, nor of predicting how delayed vocalization might be. Since communication in any form is such a vital part of human development, however, those working with young handicapped infants must remain aware of the broad nature of communication skills and must develop treatment objectives that will prepare a child to communicate through whatever means are available.

The model for communication development and the prerequisites described above provide some important guidelines for therapists and interventionists as they prepare their treatment objectives. First, *active participation* on the part of the infant is a critical component of both personal and communicative competence. To every extent possible and practical the infant should be exposed to a "contingent learning environment." That is, the environment should be responsive to his actions. The child should be observed carefully for any movements or other behaviors that might be interpreted as interest or desire so that these can be reinforced appropriately. Toys should be selected so that they can be activated in some way by the behaviors available to the child. In some cases responsive toys will have to be developed by attaching sensitive switches that the infant can operate by a slight head turn or other minimal movements.

Second, every effort should be made to promote *early communicative exchanges* between the infants and their caregivers. Despite difficulties in being able to read an infant's communicative signals, caregivers must avoid scheduling the infant's life so that she has few needs about which to communicate. Mothers should be encouraged to try to differentiate between different cries and respond accordingly; likewise, they should look for nonvocal signals of interest or desire that can be interpreted as communicative signals. Eye gaze may be particularly useful in this regard. Many developmental specialists believe that in normally developing children the mother's "attribution of communicative intent" is critical to the acquisition of communication skills.[3] That is, when the infant says "da,da,da,da,da," and the mother says, "You said daddy. Where's Daddy? There he is," she is attributing communication to the child when he may just be making sounds to please himself. The attribution, however, helps the child learn that sounds have meaning. Similarly, when an infant looks at or reaches toward a toy and the parent says, "Oh, you want the truck" she is attributing an intention to the child that may or may not be there. By the attribution and her behavior, however, she is reinforcing the child's behavior as a communicative event. The situations that lend themselves to this sort of attribution may be more limited for the severely handicapped child but we must identify those that might be useful and be less concerned about whether the child "really meant" to communicate than about teaching the child that actions can communicate.

Third, throughout all therapeutic activities thought should be given to *what behaviors might be useful as signals* or modes of communication for the child in the eventuality that speech is not possible or is insufficient for effective communication. The most efficient way to use an augmentative communication device is by direct selection, i.e., by pointing to or looking at the item to be selected. Looking is the easiest behavior to develop as a communicative signal in young handicapped children. Activities should be encouraged early in treatment that make direct gaze a reliable response. Games like peek-a-boo, or hiding toys and then showing or asking where they are, are useful for developing this skill. Communication systems which rely on pointing rather than looking, however, are more efficient. Thus, therapists should also work on skills that will promote some form of pointing, should an augmentative communication system be necessary. Such pointing might be through using the whole hand, a finger, a headstick, or a headlight. Each of these skills depends on different motor capabilities. By considering each of them in light of the child's handicaps, the therapist may be able to identify the most likely behavior a child will be able to use as a signal and develop therapeutic activities to increase the efficiency of that behavior.

Finally, the prerequisites to augmentative communication should be kept in mind as logical steps toward developing communication in handicapped infants. If the prerequisites are used as therapeutic goals for all handicapped infants, both those who will become vocal communicators and those who will have to rely on augmentative communication systems, all of these infants will be on a systematic path to communicative competence.

NOTES

1. Porter PB, Carter S, Goolsby E et al.: *Prerequisites to the Use of Augmentative Communication Systems* Chapel Hill, NC, Clinical Center for the Study of Development and Learning, University of North Carolina at Chapel Hill, 1984.

2. Vanderheiden G: Panel Discussion at the American Speech and Hearing Association, Toronto, November 1983.

3. Bruner JS: The ontogenesis of speech acts. *J Child Lang* 2: 1-19, 1975.

Psychological Assessment of the Nonvocal, Physically Handicapped Child

Nancy M. Johnson-Martin
Pamela Wolters
Shelley Stowers

SUMMARY. Although psychologists recognize the limitations of currently available tests for assessing the cognitive abilities of nonvocal, physically handicapped children, they continue to have responsibility for such assessment. Assessment is necessary to provide access to services, to determine the most appropriate learning environments and educational programs, and to develop effective augmentative communication systems. Providing a "fair" assessment is difficult. There are three approaches to such assessment: the use of currently available standardized instruments that accommodate the child's mode of response indication, the use of test modifications and the use of unique test instruments developed for this population. The problems and advantages of each of these approaches are discussed. Current best practice involves a careful consideration of the referral questions; working closely with occupational and physical therapists to assure that the child is optimally positioned and is using the most efficient mode of indication; selecting assessment instruments that will both address the specific referral questions and accommodate the child's mode of indication; remaining cautious in the interpretation of test findings; and providing frequent re-evaluations.

Since the work of Alfred Binet in France in the early 1900s, the assessment of cognitive abilities has been a major responsibility of psychologists working with children. New tests are created each year that purportedly improve the psychologist's ability to predict learning potential and to identify important strengths and weaknesses in an individual child's learning profile. An unfortunate irony, however, is that these tests are based exclusively on the skills that have been observed to emerge in normally developing children and are standardized on normal populations; yet, their primary usage is for evaluating atypical populations in which sensory, motor and cognitive abilities may emerge at different

---

Nancy M. Johnson-Martin, PhD, Head, Psychology Section, Clinical Center for the Study of Development and Learning, University of North Carolina, Chapel Hill, NC 27514.

rates and in different patterns than those observed in the normal populations. Although we can reasonably try to understand atypical children by comparing them to typical children, we must recognize that most tests of cognitive ability have been developed with an underlying assumption of intact sensory and motor systems. Children are expected to be able to manipulate objects and speak at a level commensurate with their mental capacity. When testing nonhandicapped children one rarely has to be concerned about confusing the intellectual ability with the ability to move or speak. In contrast, handicapped children may not have "normal" means of indicating their knowledge and learning abilities. Test scores, therefore, may serve only to document disabilities, not to identify abilities.

Nowhere is it more important to avoid confusing a child's output ability with his or her knowledge or understanding than in the case of the nonvocal* physically handicapped child. Most available tests of cognitive ability depend upon the person's ability to draw, write or construct with his or her hands or to speak intelligibly. Psychologists have long been aware of the limitations of these tests when applied to physically handicapped populations. In 1949 Heilman[1] noted that critical decisions were being made on the basis of the psychologist's estimates of educability but that such estimates had to be made from standardized tests that were inappropriate for the output modes of these children. Despite the recognized limitations of their tests, however, psychologists continue to have responsibility for estimating the mental capacities of the physically handicapped, and these estimates often have a major impact on the services children receive.

Although a number of efforts have been made to develop more appropriate assessment procedures since Heilman expressed his concerns, the new procedures are still inadequate for many children, the knowledge of available procedures remains limited among psychologists, and Heilman's concerns continue to be pertinent today. Almost any center that provides services to nonvocal, physically handicapped children has innumerable horror stories to tell of children who, as preschoolers, received extrapolated or computed I.Q. scores such as 9, 11, or 20 on the Slosson Intelligence Scale, the Cattell Infant Intelligence Scale, or the Bayley Scales of Infant Development. On the basis of these scores they were placed in centers for the severely retarded where stimulation was limited and they had little opportunity to hear and learn language until someone noticed their "bright eyes" or some other indication of alertness, tried to teach them, and discovered they could learn. Despite the relatively impoverished environment in which they had lived, many of these children

*The term nonvocal in this paper refers to children with no intelligible speech. Such individuals have been described by various authors as "nonvocal" or "nonverbal." Neither term is entirely accurate since the children often make some vocalizations and are frequently verbal in the sense of understanding verbal symbols and speaking some words. More recent writings in the field of augmentative communication appear to be using the term nonvocal.

have been able to demonstrate near-normal or only mildly delayed abilities when provided with appropriate education and when assessed with more appropriate procedures.

With the passage of Public Law 94-142, the Education of All Handicapped Children act in 1975, psychologists have been placed under greater pressure to provide assessments of mental abilities that do not discriminate against the child because of cultural, linguistic or specific handicapping conditions. Unfortunately, not many instruments or assessment procedures are available that can be considered "fair" for the nonvocal, physically handicapped child. Those that make provisions for the response limitations of these children frequently cover a limited age range and may include many items that are foreign to the experiences of most children who are not mobile in the environment. Yet, the need for assessment remains. The goals of this chapter are: (1) to specify the reasons a "fair" assessment of cognitive abilities is necessary, (2) to discuss some of the problems in assessment as well as the efforts that have been made to solve those problems, and (3) to describe current "best practice" as a guide for psychologists and as a reference for non-psychologists who may need to assess the adequacy of psychological evaluations done with their clients.

THE NEED FOR ADEQUATE ASSESSMENT

The Nature of the Population. The majority of nonvocal, physically handicapped children carry the diagnosis of cerebral palsy. The general belief is that a much greater incidence of mental retardation is found among those with cerebral palsy than in the normal population[2,3] and that the incidence and degree of mental retardation is related to the extent and kind of cerebral palsy.[4] Because damage to the brain is considered to be the underlying cause of cerebral palsy, it is logical to assume that it might be accompanied by cognitive deficiencies. Yet, knowing that some individuals with severe cerebral palsy are brilliant and recognizing the limitations of assessment techniques, one must be skeptical of the estimates of mental retardation that have previously appeared in the literature. If we are to understand this population and provide the necessary therapeutic and educational services, we must have more accurate estimates of the incidence of mental retardation and of any patterns of abilities that are common to individuals with cerebral palsy or to subgroups within this diagnostic category.

Access to Services and Learning Environments. In addition to simply meeting legal requirements for nonbiased assessment, an adequate assessment of the cognitive abilities of the nonvocal, physically handicapped child is necessary because, as noted above, such an assessment may have a major impact on that child's life. Decisions have been and continue to be made about the advisability of orthopedic or dental surgery and about other treatments on the basis of whether the child is thought to be cognitively capable of benefitting from such treatment. Treatments that are delayed because a child is believed to be retarded may be less effective at some later time when the determination has been made that the child is, in fact, not retarded or retarded to a lesser degree than thought initially.

A more pervasive concern is that both parental and teacher expectations are influenced by beliefs about the child's cognitive capacities. Expectations, in turn, determine the kind of experiences to which the child is exposed. If parents believe their child is retarded, they are apt to make fewer demands upon him or her and may provide a less stimulating environment in terms of the language they use and the toys and learning opportunities they provide. Teachers are likewise affected. In fact, several studies have shown a relationship between teacher expectations and pupil achievement even when pupil abilities are equated for high and low expectation groups.[5] Furthermore, in school systems administrative decisions are made about a child on the basis of his or her assessed cognitive status. In non-physically handicapped children as well as in physically handicapped children, the presence of mental retardation and the level of mental retardation determine whether the child is placed in a class where the major emphasis is on activities of daily living, pre-academic skills or academic skills; and whether the child is "mainstreamed" with normally developing children or placed in a self-contained class.

Class placement is a particularly critical issue for the nonvocal, physically handicapped child. A child who cannot speak to ask questions already has a major limitation imposed on his learning. Even experienced teachers have difficulty anticipating the questions of their pupils. Successful learning takes place as a result of children resolving their confusions through asking questions. The nonvocal child may have to depend on his talking peers to ask the questions he would like to ask in order to assimilate the information presented in the classroom. The nonvocal child with a potential for average mental ability may, therefore, be able to learn at an average rate in a normal classroom where he can hear these questions, but become functionally retarded if he spends all of his classroom time with moderately or severely retarded children who cannot conceptualize and ask questions appropriate to his level of understanding.

Planning an Appropriate Education Program. Nonvocal, physically handicapped children have a combination of abilities that may vary in severity and interact in complex ways.[6] Evidence suggests, for example, that self propelled locomotion may be an important factor in the development of spatial skills in normal children.[7] One might anticipate, therefore, that developing an awareness of space may be difficult for the child with cerebral palsy. Likewise, the inability to manipulate concrete objects may interfere with the development of number concepts. Even more than for other atypical children, accurate assessment of the strengths and weaknesses in these children is critical for effective planning of individualized education programs. Testing instruments, therefore, should not only evaluate basic cognitive skills but also examine specific skills central to educational progress.

Role in Development of an Augmentative Communication System. A careful psychological assessment of cognitive abilities is also an essential component of an augmentative communication evaluation. A child's cognitive abilities will determine his or her need for an augmentative communication system, some of the characteristics of an effective augmentative communication device, and his or her ability to use the device effectively. The psychological evaluation should provide information that will help determine the extent and nature of the child's receptive vocabulary and concepts, visual discrimination abilities, memory, and ability to learn new information. These abilities are critical factors in choosing a vocabulary for a communication device and in determining the most appropriate symbol system (objects, color picture, line drawings, words).

Augmentative communication systems vary widely in their initial complexity and in their capacity to expand to meet the growing communication needs of the user. Since the more complex systems are extraordinarily expensive, a device must be chosen that will grow with the child but does not have capacities far beyond what he or she will ever be able to use. An estimate of a child's cognitive abilities will be an important consideration in making this determination.

PROBLEMS IN ASSESSMENT

According to PL94-142, in order to provide handicapped children with the most appropriate educational services in the least restrictive environment, a full nonbiased individual evaluation is necessary to measure intellectual functioning for placement and to identify strengths and weaknesses for the development of an individual educational program. Guidelines for conducting a nonbiased assessment specify that tests and other evaluation materials should be administered in the child's primary mode of communication and validated for the specific purpose for which they are used. The evaluation should assess specific areas of educational needs as well as general intelligence; accurately reflect the child's abilities rather than reflecting any sensory, manual or speaking impairments; and evaluate all areas possibly affected by disabilities (Federal Register, 1977).[8]

Even upon casual reading of these guidelines, "nonbiased" assessment of the nonvocal, physically handicapped child appears to be a distant goal. Many nonvocal children have rudimentary communication skills at best, not a "mode of communication" in which they can be tested effectively. For the most part, tests that have been "validated" to assess intellectual functioning require speech or fine motor coordination. Little is known about all of the areas of development that might be affected by the disabilities, much less how these areas should be assessed.

In order to begin to meet the guidelines for unbiased assessment of the nonvocal, physically handicapped child, a test is required that can be administered without speech or hand manipulations. The few currently available tests that do not require such verbal or motor responses tend to measure a limited number of cognitive abilities and provide norms only for a restricted age range. Thus, deriving an accurate I.Q. score and identifying the strengths and weaknesses that are critical for developing an educational program is difficult.

Three general approaches have been used by psychologists to meet assessment requirements: (1) the use of currently available standardized assessment instruments or parts of several such instruments, (2) the modification of standardized assessment instruments, and (3) the design of unique assessment instruments, specifically for the special needs of physically handicapped children.

The Use of Standardized Assessment Instruments. The most commonly used general intelligence or mental tests are inappropriate instruments to use with nonvocal, physically handicapped children because these tests are dependent upon precise motor activity, speed of manipulation, and normal speech.[9-11] Examples of these tests are the Bayley Scales of Infant Development, the Cattell Infant Intelligence Scale, the Stanford-Binet Intelligence Test, the McCarthy Scales of Childrens Abilities and the Wechsler Intelligence Scale for Children-Revised. Scores on such tests may reflect only the effects of physical disabilities rather than providing any reasonable estimate of intellectual abilities,[10,12] however, the verbal scale of the Wechsler may be administered successfully to those few nonvocal, physically handicapped children who have adequate use of augmentative communication systems since this part of the test has no time limits.

Because of limitations in these tests, other instruments that are based on pointing and multiple choice items have been used to evaluate nonvocal, handicapped children.[13] Two examples of such tests designed for cognitive assessment are the Columbia Mental Maturity Scale[14] and the Raven's Progressive Matrices.[15] Neither require precise motor or verbal responses as the only performance requirement is to select one picture from several. They appear to have some limitations, however.[9] First, they result in a limited measure of intellectual functioning. The Columbia Mental Maturity Scale is designed for children between 3-1/2 and 10 years of age and assesses concrete (e.g., color) and abstract (e.g., category) concepts through the selection of one picture that does not belong with the rest.[14] The Raven's (ages 3 through adult) assesses both concrete and abstract concepts through the selection of a geometric pattern that completes a larger design.[15] Both assess concepts only through one type of reasoning task.[16] Neither measures the range of abilities necessary for a comprehensive understanding of mental capacity or for educational planning.

Second, the arrangement of the stimulus pictures on both tests makes accurate selection difficult for many children. On both, the pictures are too close together to enable a child with significant athetosis to point accurately or to use reliably an alternate response mode such as eye fixation. On both, the stimuli are fixed on cards making it impossible to accommodate restricted ranges of movement.

Two other examples of pictorial tests sometimes used to estimate cognitive ability are the Ammons Full Range Vocabulary Test[17] for ages 2 to adulthood and the Peabody Picture Vocabulary Test[18] for ages 2 to 18. They also require only that a child be able to select one picture from four. They are limited because they assess only vocabulary skills and share the layout problems of the Raven's and Columbia.

Despite a relatively limited age range (3 to 8 years), probably the most useful test of general cognitive ability for nonvocal, physically handicapped children is the French Pictorial Test of Intelligence (PTI).[19] This test was designed to assess abilities in both normal and handicapped children. It is composed of six subtests which assess a variety of skills considered important components of cognitive ability (vocabulary, information and comprehension, form discrimination, memory, arithmetic and similarities). Two to four pictures are located on each card and they are spaced far enough apart to accommodate imprecise hand movements and to judge eye gaze in some children. The PTI was originally standardized on a sample of normal children. Coop, Eckel and Stuck used it with cerebral palsied children and concluded it was a valid instrument for assessing their intellectual abilities.[9] Its limitations include its restricted age range and, perhaps, the questionable appropriateness of some of the items relative the usual life experiences of physically handicapped children.

Another standardized test that has promise for the evaluation of the nonvocal, physically handicapped child is the Bracken Basic Concept Scale.[20] This is not an IQ test but is well standardized and yields standard scores for children from 2 years 4 months to 8 years on a school readiness composite which includes color, letter identification, numbers, comparisons and shapes, and on other concepts important to cognitive development: direction/position, social/emotional, size, texture/material, quantity, and time/sequence. All items are administered by the examiner asking a question and the child pointing to one of several pictures to indicate an answer. This test may prove to be especially useful for assessing those concepts that are critical to educational planning. In addition, the standard scores provide a good basis for comparing a handicapped child to his or her nonhandicapped peers. In addition to the layout problems shared with other tests, a limitation of the Bracken may prove to be the complexity of the pictures. Such complexity may be a burden to the many nonvocal, physically handicapped children who have some sort of visual impairment.

The Use of Test Modifications. An alternative approach to the assessment of nonvocal, physically handicapped children is to adapt and modify the administration procedures of standardized tests.[10] Such modifications enable examiners to use selected parts of frequently used and well standardized tests measuring intellectual, achievement and language abilities in the assessment of physically handicapped children.[21]

Standardized tests, however, are meant to be administered in the exact way that they were designed.[12] When such tests are altered, each unstandardized modification depends on the judgment of the individual examiner, and adapting an item is just like creating a new test.[10] Unstandardized procedures will limit the use of the test, make difficult the use of the test in replicating research studies, destroy the test's validity,[22] and make questionable the use of test norms.[10] Before test norms are used on unstandardized procedures, a determination should be made as to how the modifications affect the performance of normal children. If the modifications significantly affect the performance of normal children, new norms should be derived[12] and validity should be evaluated by comparing the performance of a nonhandicapped group on the standard and modified versions of the test.[13]

A number of researchers have developed modifications to enable handicapped children to perform on the more frequently used standardized intelligence tests. For example, Katz[23] devised a "pointing scale method" for using the Stanford-Binet with children who could not speak or manipulate materials. The items which could be answered by pointing on forms L and M, years II through VI were grouped and prorated to obtain a mental age. Results showed that the mental age obtained by the "pointing scale method" was closely related to the mental age obtained by the standard procedure in a group of preschool cerebral palsied children. The method is limited, however, because it significantly reduces the number of test items used, results in an uneven distribution of test items at different levels, and severely handicapped children might not be able to point reliably.[21]

Sattler also modified the Stanford-Binet subtests by either altering the test stimuli or the required test response and compared the performance of handicapped and nonhandicapped children. Investigations with this procedure have suggested that the modifications are valid for assessing handicapped children with speech and motor disabilities.[13,24] In addition, he also modified the WISC-R Digit Span, Block Design and Coding subtests (using a multiple choice format). Studies indicate that only the Digit Span and Block Design subtests can be used as an alternative assessment procedure.[24]

Wamba and Marzolf used eye fixation to indicate choice of response on a modified version of the Raven's Progressive Matrices.[25] Normal children between the ages of six and eleven had similar scores under both the normal and modified conditions. In a separate study, an Etran-N response mode modification of the Progressive Matrices was compared to the normal pointing response mode by administering both modes to a group of physically disabled and a group of normal children, ages ten to thirteen years. Results indicated that the use of the modified version did not significantly affect the test scores of the normal children, but did significantly increase the scores of the physically disabled children.[12] Thus, eye gaze modifications of the Progressive Matrices would appear to be acceptable for using the standard norms, at least for children older than six years.

Many examiners involved in the assessment of physically handicapped children have modified tests by allowing children to respond by pointing, indicating yes or no as the examiner pointed, or "any other method of response the child could use . . ."[(2p 614)] Except for the studies cited above, however, little is known about the effects of modifications on obtained test results.[22] While using individualized modifications for some children may be necessary, great care must be exercised in interpreting the test results. At no time should an I.Q. be assigned to a child on the basis of these results. At best, they allow a rough estimate of the abilities and a description of what the child can do under specific circumstances. This information, however, may be quite useful in planning appropriate educational experiences.

Design of Unique Assessment Instruments. Another approach to the assessment of nonvocal, physically handicapped children is to design tests specifically for use with this population. Such tests attempt to evaluate skills in these children that are critical for their education and communication, take account of their unique life experiences, and minimize the physical aspects of the tasks. Although many such informal testing methods may be used in the field, the authors know of only one published test that was developed solely for the evaluation of the severely multiply handicapped child, the Psychological Stimulus Response (PSR) test.[26] The PSR is designed for 1- to 5-year-old multiply handicapped children or 6- to 10-year-old retarded, multiply handicapped children who cannot effectively participate in standardized testing. The stimulus response approach is designed to reduce the physical requirements of the test while tapping skills which demonstrate acquisition of concepts at various levels of intellectual development. The test consists of a Language Scale, a

Visual-Motor Scale, and a Tactile Differentiation section. Several responses are available for use by the child including vocalizations, head and facial movements, or body movements. It provides a functional age, an understanding of the child's best intake channels and most efficient response mode, and information about his or her strengths and weaknesses for educational planning.

This assessment device seems to minimize complex motor and verbal responses and to assess a wide variety of skills. It is certainly preferable to the Bayley Scales, the Cattell or the Stanford-Binet in assessing the abilities of young, nonvocal, physically handicapped children. Although it does not provide an IQ, it does provide a starting place for appropriate intervention. At the ages for which it is designed, this is probably more pertinent information; however, it has some limitations. For example, a number of visual-motor tasks still require coordinated hand movements, some response of the auditory language scale require speech, and a few of the stimulus cards display small pictures which are too close together for a reliable eye-gaze response.

The field appears to be ripe for the development of instruments that require only an indicator response (e.g., pointing, eye gaze), that assess a broad spectrum of cognitive and academic abilities, that are standardized on a nonhandicapped sample, and that are validated for both handicapped and nonhandicapped populations. Such instruments would be helpful not only for the diagnosis and educational planning of handicapped individuals, but would provide vehicles for much-needed research on the unique developmental patterns of children with speech and motor handicaps.

CURRENT BEST PRACTICE

The psychologist responsible for evaluating the cognitive and learning abilities of the nonvocal physically handicapped child can only provide adequate service with a thorough understanding of the referral questions and by collaborating with specialists in pediatric physical therapy, pediatric occupational therapy, and speech and language pathology.

Understanding the referral question. Any psychological assessment of the nonvocal, handicapped child is much more time consuming than one for the nonhandicapped child. Planning, therefore, becomes of critical importance. The first step in planning is to identify the specific purposes of the evaluation. Three basic functions of a cognitive assessment for this population are: (1) to provide an estimate of intellectual ability, i.e., to rule out mental retardation or to determine a level of retardation for placement purposes; (2) to provide information that will assist teachers in developing appropriate individual education plans, i.e., a designation of strengths and weaknesses in cognitive abilities; and (3) to provide information to aid in the development of an augmentative communication system. A referral statement, however, may not reveal how many of these functions are expected to be served by the evaluation. More frequently than not, there is a "hidden agenda." For example, many children are referred by school personnel for help in educational planning, but also with an expectation that diagnostic statements will be made about intellectual levels. Since different testing procedures and materials may be appropriate for these two purposes, the psychologist must talk to the referral source and learn of the expectations before undertaking an evaluation.

The second step is to learn as much as possible about the child's physical and communication abilities and limitations. One must know if any occupational, physical or speech therapists are working with the child and, if so, to gather as much information about the child as possible from them before making decisions about the test procedures that will be used.

Positioning. The psychologist must rely on a physical therapist for assurance that the child to be evaluated has appropriate equipment and is positioned in that equipment for optimal use of his or her body during an assessment. As noted in the chapter by Mac Neela in this volume, positioning may be a critical determinant of the ability of the child to use his or her hands to point or to use a head stick effectively. The better the child is positioned, the more reliable will be the results of the psychological evaluation.

Mode and Range of Indication. A child's mode and physical range of indication has a direct relationship to the kind of tests that are appropriate for use with that child. The psychologist, therefore, should not decide on test procedures without a prior evaluation of the child by an occupational therapist. The therapist must determine the most accurate, efficient, readable and voluntary response the child can make to interact with test materials. In order to do this, the occupational therapist must be knowledgeable about assessment instruments for this population, possible modifications of instruments, and how various modes of indication can interact with these instruments.

Many aspects of the child's neuromuscular condition must be taken into account when deciding on a mode of indication (see the chapter in this volume by Stowers and Altheide). Accuracy and range of indication on the most appropriate tests for this population require access to only two to five locations. For example, the Peabody Picture Vocabulary Test has four pictures per test item. The mode of indication selected for testing purposes should be readable 100 of the time and efficient in energy expenditure. A child may be able to access four locations using his or her hand but the movement may require such effort and time that an eye-gaze response would be more appropriate for a testing session.

The therapist should first evaluate a child's potential for using a direct selection technique. Initially, assessment of upper extremity movements, accuracy and range of movements, and the ability to isolate fingers is necessary. Grids divided into squares of different sizes can be used for the motor assessment. On each grid the child is asked to point to squares in various locations and record made of his or her accuracy and speed relative to size of grid and location on the grid. This information will enable the therapist to suggest possible modifications in test materials to facilitate the psychological assessment. An accurate readable response may be achieved by cutting apart the test pictures and arranging them in an enlarged quadrant or in some other form that accommodates the child's particular range of indication. Figure 1 shows several examples of such arrangements. From the motor assessment the therapist should also be able to provide advice regarding the best placement of test materials given the child's motor patterns (e.g., to the right or to the left of midline).

Assistive devices such as a T-bar or a hand splint with a pointer may provide the child with more discreet responses. Headstick and headlight pointers are also assistive devices that are direct selection modes of indication. If a child has had previous experience with an assistive device of this sort, it can easily be used as the response mode. Evaluation of the accuracy, range and readability of the response is still necessary, however. Assistive devices should not be utilized for testing purposes if the child is unfamiliar with them. Training sessions are required until the child is proficient in their use.

If the upper extremities and assistive devices are ruled out as the response mode, evaluation of eye gaze is necessary. Again, the accuracy, range and readability must be assessed. Use of a plexiglass sheet, approximately 24″ × 30″ with a central quadrant (5″ × 6″) cut out, enables the therapist to ascertain the viability of this response mode. The child is asked to look at the therapist through the center hole and then at various locations on the plexiglass sheet as they are pointed to by the therapist. The therapist will thereby be able to determine how readable the child's responses are and which locations increase efficiency and readability. From this assessment the therapist may suggest that the psychologist assess the child using eye-gaze system with a particular configuration of pictures. Figure 2 shows two commonly used arrangements.

If these methods of direct selection are unsuccessful, a scanning system may be necessary. If the child has a reliable yes/no response (e.g., yes = gaze up; no = head shake), the examiner can point to each picture and require a yes/no response from the child. This procedure can be very time consuming, yet may be the most appropriate mode of indication at that time. Another scanning technique is the use of a switch connected to a scanning device. A switch can require only one voluntary

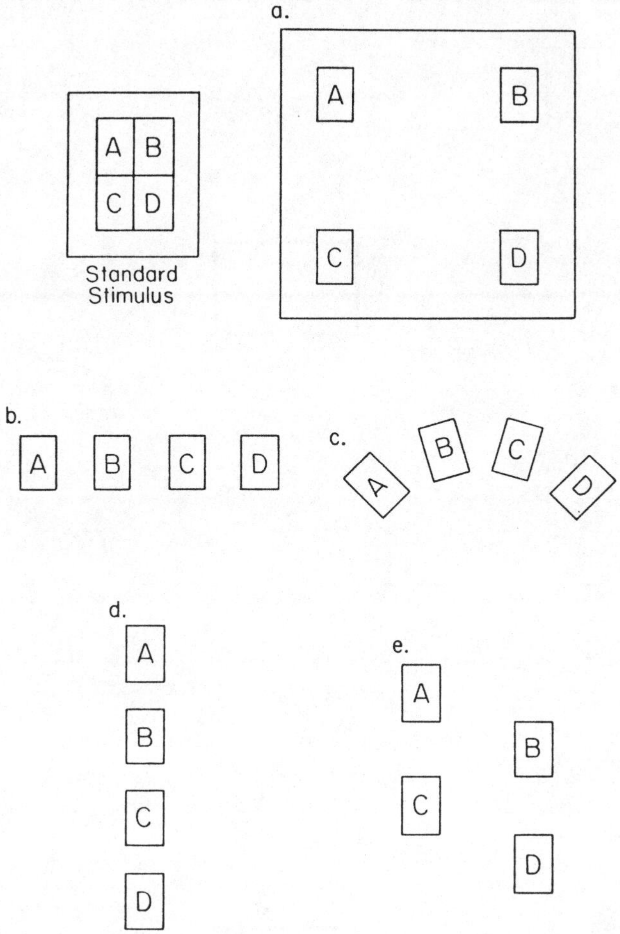

FIGURE 1. Example Arrangements of Test Stimuli to Facilitate Accurate Pointing Responses

movement and may be the only option for some severely motorically impaired children. A child must understand the switch and scanning process and have had previous experience using such a system before being asked to use it in a testing session.

Selection of Assessment Procedures. The psychologist's perception of the specific referral questions necessarily determines which procedure will be used in the psychological evaluation. If the diagnosis of mental ability is a critical issue for educational placement or for other major decisions, the psychologist must choose a standardized test and give it in as standard a way as possible. Any modifications that are made in the test

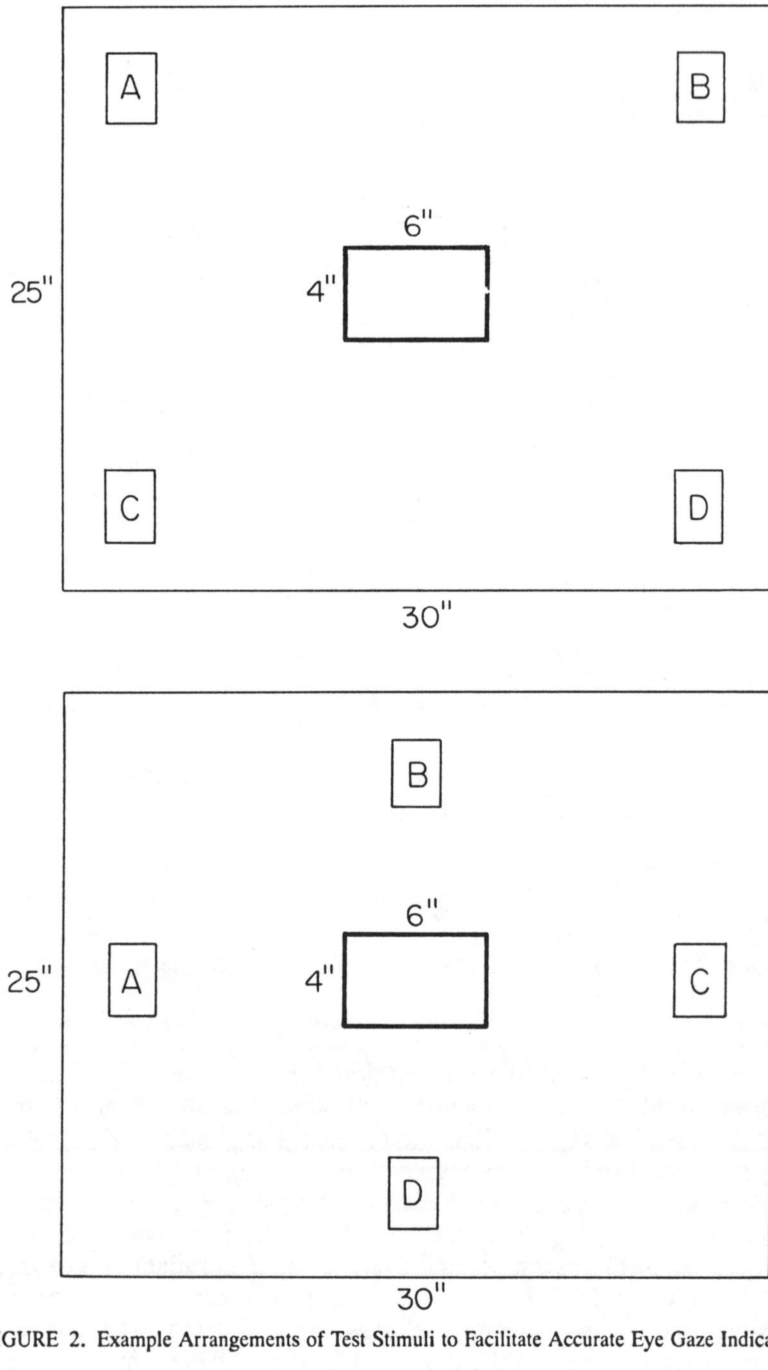

FIGURE 2. Example Arrangements of Test Stimuli to Facilitate Accurate Eye Gaze Indication

procedure must be specified and reported carefully and cautions must be applied to the interpretation of the test result. For purposes of educational planning, however, procedures can be chosen that are not standardized but that will identify skills relevant to academic success. An educational specialist should be called upon to assess the child who is already reading and doing other academic work but who is experiencing specific learning difficulties. The psychologist can be effective, however, in evaluating basic readiness skills such as form, letter and word discrimination, general information, concepts, listening comprehension and number concepts. Materials may be drawn from existing tests and the response requirements modified with impunity if the issue is what the child can do given sufficient latitude in responding rather than identifying some standard readiness or grade score.

If one of the goals for the evaluation is to provide assistance in planning an augmentative communication system, the psychologist should work closely with the speech and language specialist in determining what kinds of information would be most useful from the psychological evaluation. The language specialist may already have a good assessment of the child's vocabulary and grammatical understanding. In such a case, the psychologist's evaluation may need to focus on the range of concepts the child understands, the range of information about which he or she may wish to communicate, the child's ability to discriminate visually the symbols that might be used in a communication system, or the child's rate of learning a simple symbol system. Standardized procedures are not necessary for obtaining these sorts of information; the psychologist must rely on his or her ingenuity in adapting and designing materials.

SUMMARY

The psychological evaluation of the nonvocal, physically handicapped child is a special challenge to the psychologist. These children do not have the speech and fine motor skills that are normally prerequisites for a valid determination of intellectual and academic abilities. The psychologist, therefore, must remain humble about his or her limitations and the limitations of the available assessment instruments. Psychologists, however, must also recognize the assessment needs of this population and work toward meeting these needs in a highly professional manner. Thoughtful collaboration with other professionals who have knowledge of these children, careful planning of assessment procedures to meet specified goals, cautious interpretation of test results, and reassessment at regular intervals will lead to the best psychological services for these children and to continued development of better assessment procedures for the future.

NOTES

1. Heilman AE: Appraisal of abilities of the cerebral palsied child. *Am J Ment Defic* 53: 606-609, 1949.

2. Miller E, Rosenfeld GB: The psychologic evaluation of children with cerebral palsy and its implications in treatment. *Pediatrics* 41:613-621, 1952.

3. Fisch, CB, Yang DC, Yuin C, et al.: Intellectual development of children with cerebral palsy, in Baum D (ed): Annual Meeting of the American Academy for Cerebral Palsy and Developmental Medicine. *Dev Med Child Neurol* 21:109-122, 1979.

4. Davies PA, Drillien CM, Foley J. et al.: Cerebral Palsy, in Drillien CM, Drummond NB (eds): *Neurodevelopmental Problems in Early Childhood: Assessment and Management*. Oxford, Blackwell Scientific Publications, 1977.

5. Rosenthal R, Jacobson L: Self-fulfilling prophecies in the classroom: Teachers' expectations as unintended determinants of pupils' intellectual competence, in Deutsch M, Katz I, Jensen AR (eds): *Social Class, Race and Psychological Development*. New York, Holt Rinehart and Winston, 1968.

6. Wolf JM, Anderson RM: *The Multiply Handicapped Child*. Springfield, IL, Charles C Thomas, 1969.

7. Campos JJ, Berthanal BI: The importance of self-produced locomotion in infancy. *Infant Mental Health Journal* 5:160-171, 1984.

8. Education of handicapped children, implementation of part B of the Education of the Handicapped act. *Federal Register* 42:42473-42518 (August 23) 1977.

9. Coop RH, Eckel E, Stuck GB: An assessment of the Pictorial Test of Intelligence with young cerebral palsied children. *Dev Med Child Neurol*17:287-292, 1975.

10. Sattler JM, Tozier LL: A review of intelligence test modifications used with cerebral palsied and other handicapped groups. *J Spec Ed* 4:391-398, 1970.

11. Blum LH, Burgemeister B, Lorge I: Trends in estimating the mental maturity of the cerebral palsied child. *Excep Child* 17:174-177, 1951.

12. Brown RJ, McMullen P: An unbiased response mode for assessing intellectual ability in normal and physically disabled children. *Clin Neuropsychol* 4:51-56, 1982.

13. Barnett AJ: Defining an assessment of the child with cerebral palsy. *Psychol Sch*19:160-165, 1982.

14. Burgemeister B, Blum LH, Lorge I: *Columbia Mental Maturity Scale*. Yonkers on the Hudson, NY, World Book Co, 1954.

15. Raven JC. *Standard Progressive Matrices*. London, HK Lewis and Co. Ltd, 1958.

16. Nicholson C: Correlations among CMMS, PVT, RCPM for cerebral palsied children. *Percept Mot Skills* 30:715-718, 1970.

17. Ammons RB, Ammons HS: *The Full-range Picture Vocabulary Test*. New Orleans, RB Ammons, 1948.

18. Dunn LM, Dunn LM: *Peabody Picture Vocabulary Test-Revised*. Circle Pines, MN, American Guidance Service, 1981.

19. French JL: *Pictorial Test of Intelligence*. Boston, Houghton Mifflin Co, 1964.

20. Bracken BA: *Bracken Basic Concept Scale*. Columbus, OH, Charles E. Merrill Publishing Co, 1984.

21. Katz E: The pointing scale method: A modification of the Stanford-Binet procedure for use with cerebral palsied children. *Am J Ment Defic* 60:838-842, 1956.

22. Bragman R: Review of test instructions for deaf children. *Am Ann Deaf* 127:337-346, 1982.

23. Katz E: The "pointing modification" of the revised Stanford-Binet Intelligence Scales, forms L and M, years II through VI: A report of research in progress. *Am J Ment Defic* 62: 698-707, 1958.

24. Harrington RG: A review of Sattler's modifications of standard intelligence tests for use with handicapped children. *Sch Psychol Digest* 8:296-302, 1979.

25. Wamba DF, Marzolf SS: Use of eye movements as a response indicator in testing the physically handicapped. *J Clin Psychol* 11:405-407, 1955.

26. Mullen EM: *Psychological S-R Evaluation for Severely Multiply Handicapped Children*. East Providence, RI, Meeting Street School, 1977.

An Overview of Therapeutic Positioning for Multiply-Handicapped Persons, Including Augmentative Communication Users

Jane C. Mac Neela

SUMMARY. The body of literature related to adaptive equipment for positioning clients with neuro-musculoskeletal disorders has expanded slowly since the early 1970s. Much of this literature describes custom solutions to positioning problems for individual clients with cerebral palsy. Papers addressing the positioning needs for augmentative communication users remain sparse and superficial in scope. Furthermore, the literature on adaptive equipment solutions is substantially limited to clinicians' perceptions and theoretical premises of the effectiveness of positioning devices. Few formal studies of the effects of positioning have been reported, and none of the studies have addressed the relationship of body positioning to the use of augmentative communication devices.

The purpose of this paper is to provide a review of the literature devoted to formal studies and guidelines for the use of therapeutic positioning for clients with multiple physical needs. Considerations for employing seating and positioning systems with clients using augmentative or alternative means of communication will also be addressed.

Clinicians and authors who serve multiply-handicapped children and adults with augmentative communication needs are aware of the importance of therapeutic positioning as it relates to effective means of expression. Klein commented that the client who requires an elaborate augmentative communication system is likely to be severely physically handicapped and have difficulty maintaining proper sitting posture.[1]

Jane C. Mac Neela, LPT, is a staff physical therapist at the Clinical Center for the Study of Development and Learning, University of North Carolina at Chapel Hill and a candidate for the Master of Science degree in Medical Allied Health Professions with a major in Physical Therapy (Pediatrics) at the University of North Carolina at Chapel Hill. Her graduate work is supported in part by Grant 149, Postgraduate Programs in Maternal and Child Health Care, Bureau of Health Care Delivery and Assistance, Health Resources and Services Administration, USPHS, DHHS. Reprint requests should be addressed to the author at Clinical Center for the Study of Development and Learning, BSRC-220H, University of North Carolina at Chapel Hill, Chapel Hill, NC 27514.

Schurman added that sitting posture was especially important for the child using a headstick-pointing method to access a communication system, in that extraneous movement of the trunk and arms diminished the effective range of headstick-pointing by disturbing trunk balance.[2]

Despite the acknowldgement that body alignment is an important component for clients using augmentative communication systems, little has been written on this topic. Several authors have addressed this issue very briefly, without offering practical guidelines for integrating therapeutic positioning with communication devices.[1-4] No formal studies have addressed the relationship between optimal body alignment and use of augmentative communication devices.

Although supportive empirical data are lacking, the literature suggests that most clinicians believe therapeutic positioning plays an integral role in the physically handicapped client's effective use of an augmentative communication device. Many centers serving handicapped clients offer an interdisciplinary staff and facilities for prescription, fabrication and adaptation of therapeutic positioning components, often interfaced with augmentative communication devices. Manufacturers of adaptive equipment have gradually expanded their product lines to include more versatile positioning components which promote improved function and comfort for these persons with multiple needs. These factors suggest that, in general, clinicians identify a positive relationship between therapeutic positioning and optimal functional use of augmentative communication systems for clients with significant physical deficits.

THERAPEUTIC POSITIONING AS IT RELATES TO FUNCTION

Much of the literature addressing therapeutic positioning describes the effects of improved alignment in terms of enhanced functional capabilities. If we assume that the use of communication devices is dependent on functional ability, improved body alignment could increase a given client's communicative skills, whether he or she accesses a device via upper extremity pointing, use of a head-stick/light, or any other mode employing a body part.

Proposed Benefits and Purposes for Therapeutic Positioning

Many reasons for positioning clients having motor impairments have been reported in the literature. Among these various claims are proposed benefits for the musculoskeletal, cardio-respiratory, and nervous systems, in addition to improved functional abilities and ease of client care by others. The reader is encouraged to critique these claims carefully, giving consideration to the limited or absent proof for each postulate as offered in the subsequent literature review section of this paper.

The following list of these purposes is varied and quite extensive in scope. These have been grouped into two major sections: functionally and physiologically-based purposes. Postulates stated by individual authors may overlap those of others; wherever some discrepancy was noted, these related principles were cited separately for purposes of clarity.

The reasons for therapeutic positioning noted within this literature review included:

A. *Functional Purposes*:

1. to provide physical support/stability which promotes functional improvements [5]
2. to normalize muscle tone and facilitate more normal movement patterns, maximizing function with minimal movement pathology [5,6]
3. to control abnormal movement patterns[7]
4. to facilitate components of normal movement in a developmental sequence by incorporating proper weight-bearing, weight shifting, rotation, and righting reactions [4-6]
5. to promote more independent mobility [4,5,7-10]
6. to provide comfort and relaxation in a more upright position[3,6,7,8,10,11]
7. to allow maximal upper limb function[6,10-12]
8. to facilitate communication via well-controlled upright positioning[3,7,8,12]
9. to facilitate physical and occupational therapy by providing upright positions suitable for strengthening and coordination exercises[7]
10. to faciliate recreational and social activities, enhanced by more upright positioning[3,4,7,9]
11. to promote the psychological benefits of the upright position by placing clients in more socially acceptable, "less handicapped" postures [4,7]
12. to facilitate education via upright positioning in the classroom[3,7,12]
13. to facilitate vocational activities[7]
14. to facilitate independence in self-care activities [4,7]
15. to facilitate nursing care (feeding, toileting, bathing the upper body) via upright alignment[7,12]
16. to allow ease of transportation of clients to and from schools, developmental centers, and community centers, by parents and attendants[10,11,12]

B. *Physiologic Purposes*:

1. to prevent or correct joint contractures and skeletal deformities, and increase range of motion[5-8,10,11,13]
2. to facilitate the sensation of good body alignment[4,5]
3. to facilitate respiratory gas exchange[7]

4. to facilitate cardiac muscle function[7]
5. to promote general health and resistance to infection[7]

Although many of these statements seem to be theoretically sound, little proof of these premises has been provided via formal studies documented in the literature. Furthermore, the benefits of therapeutic positioning for oral or augmented communication have not been validated.

Formal Studies of Therapeutic Positioning

The practice of therapeutic positioning and seating is relatively recent in origin, and the literature on this topic seems to cover several areas. The most popular approach to documentation on this issue has been the case report method, citing custom-fitted solutions to individual client's needs. Although these are helpful in sharing creative solutions to positioning problems, more formal studies of the effectiveness of positioning are needed. This section provides a review of the available formal studies related to therapeutic positioning. Readers are encouraged to consider that these studies contain the only evidence provided for validation of the aforementioned purposes for therapeutic positioning.

Within this review, the first three studies address functional gains following positioning intervention. The next two papers focus on the issue of therapeutic positioning applied to improve head control during feeding programs. The last two studies address more physiologic aspects of therapeutic positioning, evaluating the effects on pulmonary function and spasticity, respectively.

Hulme and associates[14] described a rural, home-based model for provision of adaptive equipment to physically-handicapped clients throughout the state of Montana. Although the purpose of this paper was to describe the implementation of the project, the authors also cited several examples of the effectiveness of their interventions. These results were incidentally described in functional terms for individual clients, including improvements in head and trunk control, sucking and swallowing ability, finger feeding, and increased frequency and ease of mobility out of the home environment. Use of an objective rating scale for determining these improvements was not apparent.

In a follow-up study, Hulme and colleagues[15] reported the perceived functional benefits for clients receiving adaptive equipment. By administering a post-hoc written questionnaire to clients' caretakers, the investigators documented improvement in ability of 65.5% of the subjects to sit upright without leaning. Sitting tolerance also increased from a mean interval of 3-4 hours to a mean interval of 4-5 hours, following equipment intervention. Significant improvement was reported for eating manner, drinking manner, and ability to reach for and grasp an object. Also cited were improved independence in toileting, mobility in the home environment, and access to the community environment. The inter-relationship between adaptive seating and augmentative communication devices was not described in this functional review. The authors acknowledged that the documented functional improvements could not be attributed to adaptive equipment intervention alone, as many of the clients were concurrently involved in therapeutic training programs for motor and sensory skills, feeding, and upright mobility.

Trefler and co-workers[16] completed a similar study to examine the effects of establishing a delivery program to provide ten physically-handicapped students with adaptive equipment for seating, communication, mobility, and personal care. Analysis of serial measures taken during an 18-month period revealed a significant increase to seven hours, for mean duration of upright head and trunk alignment, when eight of the students were positioned in their respective "therapeutic seating systems." Significant improvement in gross arm control was also reported for the therapeutic seating condition. Progress in feeding skills was reported for students who received technical feeding aids. Influence of therapeutic seating on feeding skills was not discussed. The authors described a training program for improving motor skills required to operate the control switches (e.g., arm-slot control requiring only a gross placement of the arm within 1 of 5 "troughs," and single-switch control requiring more accurate placement and activation by arm pressure on a single paddle) for powered technical aids. The trained students demonstrated two to four times more proficiency in operating two devices accessed by these two switches. Although the authors mentioned the provision of augmentative communication devices for some of the subjects in this study, the relationship between therapeutic positioning and use of such communication units was not addressed. The functional transfer of arm-placement training to implementation with communication devices was similarly not reported. Also, the authors did not clarify whether or not the students were positioned in their respective therapeutic seating systems during the arm-placement training, feeding training, and power wheelchair training.

O'Brien and Tsurumi[17] compared head-righting abilities as an effect of sitting in an adapted wheelchair versus semi-prone positioning on a prone support device (angled 30 degrees from the horizontal). Each of the 26 clients' wheelchairs had been custom-designed and fabricated "to bring the individual client into the best possible body alignment in the seated position."[17(p675)] Body alignment to a given standard (e.g., back-rest reclined 10° from the vertical, with seat/back-rest angle at 10°/90°) was not described. The authors stated that none of the subjects used a formal communication mode, either verbal or non-verbal. Mercury head switches were used to determine the range of head movement during the two test conditions; frequency and duration of head positioning within a predetermined 30° range was measured. In order to stimulate headrighting, food was presented every 15 seconds and the subject was fed by an examiner. Each subject participated in one session of prone and sitting testing, each condition lasting 7 and 10 minutes, respectively. The authors concluded that frequentcy and duration of head-righting while sitting in an adapted wheelchair was no different from frequency and duration of head-righting while semi-prone on a positioning device. Longer duration of head-righting was significantly correlated with those clients who had more skilled wheelchair mobility. Comparison of head-righting before and after receipt of adaptive seating components was not addressed. Frequency and duration of spontaneous head-righting without food stimulus was not reported.

Lee and co-workers[18] described a single case study of the effect of midline head positioning on the incidence of the asymmetrical tonic neck reflex (ATNR). The authors introduced a midline-stabilizing foam headpiece into the feeding seat used by an 11.5 year-old profoundly retarded female with cerebral palsy. For an initial period of 7 days, baseline frequency of ATNR activity was recorded during feeding. The headpiece was cut away or scooped out gradually during 12 successive "treatment" sessions, each time the examiner(s) had noted no ATNR activity during three successive lunch periods. In addition, quality of biting was scored, with a "correct" bite consisting of one bite of food placed in the subject's mouth without evidence of a bite reflex occurring. By the end of the intervention period (88 days), the client could consistently demonstrate the "correct" bite pattern during 100% of the lunch period. On Day 70, the foam headpiece had been removed and the client maintained her new skills during a 19-day trial period. The authors concluded that gradual withdrawal of the head support could be considered an effective approach to reducing abnormal reflex posturing, but additional studies were indicated to clarify the exact mechanism by which these changes had been effected. Endurance and carry-over of this newly acquired head control skill to non-lunch periods (e.g., throughout the day) were not addressed.

Nwaobi and Smith[19] studied the effect of adaptive seating on the pulmonary function of nine children diagnosed as having cerebral palsy. Measurements of vital capacity, forced expiratory volume, and end of tidal volume were taken for each subject, under two conditions; seated in a standard wheelchair with and without adapted positioning components. The three pulmonary parameters showed mean increases of 51.6 to 57.7% when the clients were positioned in the wheelchair with the adaptive inserts. The authors credited these statistically significant improvements in pulmonary function to the assisted upright alignment of the neck, thorax, and abdomen, as provided by the positioning components.

Nwaobi and colleagues[20] examined the electromyographic (EMG) activity of the (lumbar) erector spinae muscles at various sitting angles, in 11 children diagnosed as having spastic cerebral palsy. The test chair was adjusted to standardized alignment criteria for each child's body proportions. The examiners noted that EMG activity (as measured by mean action potential counts) was least when the seat/backrest angle was 0°/90° (reference was horizontal). Highest EMG activity was noted at seat/backrest angles of 0°/75°, followed by lesser activity at 15°/120° and 0°/120° respectively. Action potential counts were lower in the 0° seat angle than in the 15° seat surface inclination. The authors cited a previously unpublished study in which Nwaobi and Cusick[21] determined that EMG activity in the hip adductor muscles was least at the 15°/90° seat/backrest position, compared with a variety of other positions examined. Nwaobi and colleagues[20] cited limitations of their study with regard to the degree of variability in EMG activity among subjects. They surmised that this was related to the severity of the motor impairment for each subject and suggested use of a clinical classification system for subject selection in future studies. Functional activities (including use of augmentative communication devices) at various seat/backrest angles were not addressed.

In summary, the body of literature addressing the topic of therapeutic seating and positioning remains very limited, with notable deficiency in documentation of needs and recommendations for clients using alternative communication systems. The available papers, however, can be very useful to the clinician. The outcomes of the seven formal studies certainly lend some support to several of the purposes which we associate with therapeutic positioning. The variability in approaches and lack of replication, however, impose limits on the strength of these claims. Facilities which specialize in the delivery of therapeutic positioning services should encourage implementation of clinical studies designed to examine the validity of these beliefs, especially as they relate to functional use of augmented communication devices.

THE NEED FOR A MORE DEFINITIVE APPROACH TO THERAPEUTIC POSITIONING

In view of the fact that we have little evidence of the effects of therapeutic positioning, and considering the variety of approaches with which clinicians evaluate postural alignment in multiply-handicapped clients, this author believes that a more definitive approach to positioning intervention is needed. At present, clinicians' knowledge and application of the principles of biomechanics, optimal postural alignment, and perceived benefits of therapeutic positioning appears to be quite varied. The limitations of therapeutic positioning intervention have not been studied, and clinicians and researchers have not yet defined those aspects about which we need further information. Since the practice of providing therapeutic positioning is a recently evolved specialty, most therapists have learned these skills during their clinical experiences. It is unlikely that positioning training programs have been developed for inclusion within the academic curricula of university programs in physical or occupational therapy. In essence, we have not yet determined a standard approach to therapeutic positioning, identifying the formal evaluation components which should be included, nor do we have agreement regarding optimal alignment criteria for promoting specific functional capabilities in multiply-handicapped individuals. With the exception of Heinrich's chapter on materials and fabrication techniques,[22] indications and contraindications for selecting specific materials and components are not clear, although several authors have offered opinions in this regard based on their clinical experiences.[5,6,11,23,24] For a more comprehensive, mechanical, and functional review of positioning materials, readers are referred to Heinrich's engineering approach to the assessment of these components.[22]

In addition to the needs for research of current practices as cited above, a second approach to formal investigation of therapeutic positioning is suggested in the area of product development and testing. The variety of materials and approaches to positioning have increased during recent years, partially in response to needs identified by therapists working in this area of patient care.[23] Custom-molding, vacuum-fitting, and other methods of aligning clients with musculoskeletal deficits have been developed by several companies. In addition, equipment vendors have begun to offer more adaptive services by customizing standard wheelchair components for individual patients, as requested by physicians and therapists. Although these improvements in service delivery have provided significant increases in the options which a given client may obtain, continued development and *testing* of therapeutic positioning components and materials is needed. Particular attention should be devoted to identifying those positioning components and materials which facilitate clients' functional capabilities, including the access and operation of augmentative communication devices.

Traditionally, therapists have been relied upon to determine the specific adaptations to align their clients for wheelchair sitting and other forms of positioning. This is often done in consultation with a physician. Although therapists and physicians are knowledgeable about musculoskeletal development and functioning, other professionals possess the assessment skills and knowledge of biomechanical principles which are exerted through positioning. In view of the introduction of new materials and more versatile components into this market of positioning equipment, engaging the consultative services of biomedical or rehabilitation engineers seems appropriate. As a related consideration, the field of ergonomics (the application of scientific principles to evaluating the most efficient use of human energy for given tasks[25,26]) may offer another approach to evaluating optimal positioning for such clients. This field is relatively new and its scope of practice seems to have been limited to evaluation and remediation of environmental conditions affecting able-bodied workers in their individual job settings. The same concerns of muscular fatigue, postural alignment, and preventing injury are applicable to handicapped persons, particularly for those individuals who must substitute compensatory movement patterns for functional activities which are otherwise impossible (e.g., using the neck muscles for the "fine motor" task of accessing a communication unit via a head-stick/light). Ergonometric analysis of a handicapped individual's postural and movement patterns while using an augmentative communication device might provide important information regarding selection of the most efficient orientation of the client and the communication unit. Although the application of ergonomic assessment may be appropriate for determining the optimal functional position for a given client's ability to operate an augmentative communication device, the fact that the physically handicapped person's neuro-musculoskeletal system is inherently different from normal should not be overlooked.

Finally, a more precise approach to the application of positioning components should be considered. Many clinicians are familiar with the degree and specificity of forces which an orthotist incorporates into a total contact brace for scoliosis, by using palpation and radiography in this process. We appear to be far less precise when we apply the same principles through selection and placement of corresponding components for therapeutic wheelchair seating. For example, how often do we use radiography and repeated palpation and fittings in determining the exact location of the apex of a scoliotic curve, when specifying the final placement for lateral trunk supports attached to a wheelchair? Do we consistently apply biomechanical forces in a *systematic* manner to stabilize deformities? Lack of such precision may contribute to error in aligning clients with physical deficits. Additional sources of error or lack of specificity in applying external supports for therapeutic positioning include:

1. limitations of "one size fits all" or "stock" components and adaptations offered by wheelchair manufacturers;
2. limited access to custom-fitting services and trained personnel at regional rehabilitation and vending facilities specializing in therapeutic positioning;
3. numerous caretakers (with varying degrees of training in therapeutic positioning) involved in re-positioning the client throughout the day;
4. errors in re-applying removable or adjustable components of the positioning system, including loss or misplacement of detachable parts; and
5. inability of the client to instruct caretakers in proper techniques for adjusting positioning when applied incorrectly.

Increased precision and a more definitive approach to applying forces for therapeutic positioning would contribute reliability to this process, in addition to providing a more standardized base from which we could infer the effects of this intervention. Perhaps the use of radiography before and after positioning (e.g., as done with scoliosis bracing) would indicate the degree of correction gained from providing external supports to specific body parts.

In an effort to increase the availability of more adaptable materials and components for positioning, clinicians who specialize in this practice might convey specific needs, ideas, and problems to product manufacturers and facilities which offer positioning services. With regard to improving compliance of caretakers involved in re-positioning these clients, Lattimore and colleagues recommended that very specific training procedures and follow-up are necessary, including a written checklist which itemizes each positioning component for a given client.[27]

In general, reducing sources of error and increasing the precision of the positioning process is an important prerequisite for contributing evidence to prove the premises for this clinical practice.

ADDITIONAL CONSIDERATIONS REGARDING THERAPEUTIC POSITIONING

Biomechanical Principles

In addition to formal studies of therapeutic positioning, several authors have focused attention on the biomechanical principles which are incorporated into this clinical practice.

Therapeutic positioning involves the biomechanical application of forces such as compression, distraction, and shearing.[28] These forces, when acting externally on a body, are called loads. The internal forces within the structure responding to these loads are called reaction stresses. Each load or stress is specified by four distinguishing descriptors: magnitude, line of application (the action line), direction (toward or away from the structure upon which it acts), and point of application. *Pressure*, which is an important aspect of force, indicates how the force is distributed over an area. In addition, the "give" or yield of the material contacting and supporting the body surfaces is a primary factor in avoiding dangerous effects of continuous pressure.[28,29]

Nwaobi, in his excellent chapter titled *Biomechanics of Seating*,[28] pointed to the complexity and precision of these combined forces required to stabilize a spinal curve or pelvic deformity when using positioning components in a therapeutic seating system. As an example of such seating, he described the degree of refinement needed in applying the three point force system used in controlling spinal alignment for scoliosis. He stated that proportional force pads should be placed at the apex of the curve, with specified opposing forces placed at strategic points.[28]

Another factor which he addressed was the alignment of the lumbar spine in sitting. Some clinicians have specified that lumbar lordosis is desirable when re-aligning the deviated spine, because the lumbar facet joints engage and tighten in extension and provide stability to the superincumbent vertebrae.[30,31] Although lumbar lordosis is the natural alignment for the upright individual, it may be more facilitatory to abnormal extensor movement patterns in clients who are dominated by these patterns. Nwaobi described the adjustment of the normal pelvis and spine when the sitting posture is assumed: the psoas muscles relax; the hamstring and hip extensor muscles become tight; and the pelvis assumes a posterior tilt, reversing the lumbar lordosis. He added that, when the lumbar spine reverses to a more flexed alignment, the line of gravity moves anterior to the vertebral joints, increasing the lever arm of the force of gravity. The level of activity in the lumbar extensor muscles consequently increases in order to maintain equilibrium in the spine. Nwaobi suggested that this kyphotic position of the lumbar spine may not be the best position for the client who demonstrates significant extensor spasticity. Instead, promoting lumbar lordosis will alter the gravity line and reduce the level of extensor muscle activity required to maintain equilibrium.[28]

As a separate consideration, Ogden added that the child's spine remained more mobile than the adult's spine, and that externally-applied forces would be more easily dissipated over a greater number of segments.[32] This would reinforce the need for absolute accuracy in applying loads to stabilize or correct a specified skeletal deviation in the spine. Similarly, LeVeau and Bernhardt emphasized the need to consider critical periods of rapid growth in children, when skeletal tissue could be most susceptible to the forces placed upon it.[33]

Since therapeutic seating involves the application of biomechanical forces to promote functional upright posture, the biomechanical components of joint and muscle flexibility and skeletal alignment must be carefully assessed. Norkin and Levangie stated that the body may act as a closed kinematic chain, in that repositioning of one segment will influence adjacent segments, resulting in re-distribution of normal compressive stresses and of normal shear stresses. They addressed the issue of lumbar-pelvic rhythm, stating that a restriction of motion at either the lumbar spine or at the hip joints will disturb this rhythm, and that the integration of motion of the pelvis with the motion of the spine will affect the mobility and flexibility of the total vertebral column.[34] Bohannon and colleagues studied the lumbo-pelvic rhythm in a small sample of 17 normal subjects, and they determined that pelvic motion is highly correlated with active and passive hip flexion, to the extent that pelvic rotation accounts for 25-33 percent of total hip flexion movement. They also acknowledged that pelvic and hip mobility are interrelated such that any abnormality affecting one component may affect the total hip flexion movement.[35] Their findings suggested that clinicians should be aware of the significant contribution of pelvic motion to hip flexion movement, especially from a measurement standpoint.

When assessing patients for therapeutic positioning intervention, passive joint ranges of motion should be measured with precision, giving special attention to hip joint mobility compared to pelvic motion. To examine this relationship, the client is positioned in supine and the pelvis must be *stabilized* while the clinician passively moves one leg at a time into hip flexion and monitors for pelvic movement by holding the ipsilateral ilium with his or her other hand. This is critical for clients who may be considered as candidates for a "wedge"-type seat which requires more than 90° of hip flexion (seat/backrest angle less than 90°, with seat usually rotated 10-15° up from the horizontal). If hip flexion mobility is inadequate, the missing range will be taken up by the pelvis, which will rotate toward a posterior tilt (symphysis up) and facilitate lumbar kyphosis. According to this author's clinical experiences, skin breakdown or pressure over the posterior bony prominences of the pelvis or lumbar spine is not uncommon when passive hip flexion mobility is inadequate and very flexed seating angles are sought. In addition, as Nwaobi has described, lumbar kyphosis may be undesirable for clients who demonstrate significant extensor spasticity since these muscles may be facilitated to contract more vigorously in this position.[28] Finally, vertebral stability of the lumbar spine (and super-incumbent segments) may be diminished when it is aligned in flexion, owing to the orientation of the lumbar facet joints.[30,31]

Clinicians must be aware of the compensatory reactions which may occur when one musculoskeletal segment is adjusted against another segment. Keeping in mind the biomechanical forces of compression, shearing, and distraction, we may impose undesirable postural adjustments which may contribute to deformity, when we apply forces to align segments which cannot withstand the same. The following section of this paper provides collected guidelines for therapeutic positioning as offered by a variety of occupational and physical therapists and several other clinicians who have written on this subject. With regard to applying these guidelines to individual patients, clinicians should be aware of the variation among these authors' opinions and suggestions for positioning (e.g., debate over lumbar kyphosis versus lordosis for stability of the superincumbent spine). Hopefully, future studies will clarify discrepant points from the literature, so that therapists and other health professionals can apply objective postural alignment criteria to assessment and positioning intervention for clients with identified biomechanical or musculoskeletal limitations and needs.

CLINICAL GUIDELINES FROM THE LITERATURE: POSITIONING THE HANDICAPPED CLIENT

Various guidelines for positioning physically-compromised clients in optimal seating alignment have been suggested by several clinicians.[3,8,11,36,37] These guidelines are summarized in Table 1. In general, these authors agreed that the hips, knees, and ankles should be positioned as close to 90 degrees (each), as possible, and the pelvis should be centered in midline. Trefler and colleagues[37] and Trefler and Taylor[8] commented that the trunk should approximate a vertical midline alignment whenever possible. Motloch, Trefler and colleagues, Hacker, and Trefler and Taylor recommended that the head should be held in midline-vertical position, without stimulation over the occipital area.[3,8,11,37] The position of the upper extremities was not addressed by most of these (and other) authors.

Trefler and Taylor[8] and Ward[6] agreed that the pelvis should be the first body part to be positioned, in conjunction with the lower extremities. The trunk should be aligned on that "base" and, last, the position of the head and upper extremities should be addressed.

McGee identified the tendency for clinicians to position a severely-involved client in a rigid seating-support system, thereby diminishing his or her opportunity to use body control for function. She suggested that each system should provide opportunities for the client to have full support when necessary, but also permit active postural control by the client, whenever appropriate.[38] Wilson agreed that adaptive equipment should not restrict the child's movements, but rather increase the child's possibilities to practice and use movements he or she is developing.[4] McGee[38] concurred with Trefler and Taylor[8] and Ward[6] regarding the importance of positioning the pelvis and lower body as a "base." She stated that firm support of the trunk and legs was important for these severelyinvolved clients, as they often use head, neck, shoulders, and arms to initiate functional movements.[38]

In summary, therapeutic positioning is considered to be an important intervention strategy used by clinicians who manage clients with musculoskeletal disorders. Loose guidelines for seating these clients have been offered by a number of authors, based on their clinical experiences and observations.[3,6,8,9,11,28,36-38] Suggestions for positioning clients in alternative devices are also available,[6] although these are less specific in terms of alignment criteria. According to this review of the literature, guidelines for positioning the upper extremities have not been specified for clients

TABLE 1. Guidelines for Positioning

	HEAD	UPPER LIMBS	TRUNK	HIPS	KNEES	ANKLES & FEET	MATERIALS
Trefler and Taylor (1984)	held in midline with minimum support needed; avoid stimulation over occiput	encourage shoulder protraction	held in midline using lateral trunk supports as needed; 3-point pressure applied for scoliotic curves; vertical trunk alignment preferred; reclined angles determined on an individual basis for clients with poor trunk control	pelvis and hips held in midline; flexing the hips past 90° encourages a more relaxed, abducted posture for clients with significant extensor tone; hips should be "slightly abducted"	knees and ankles should be at 90° unless precluded by severe extensor tone or fixed orthopedic deformities; feet should always be well supported to prevent deformity and maintain appropriate knee and ankle angles; dorsiflexing ankles slightly may help to reduce both clonus and extensor tone		lapbelt should be snug across the hips, mounted at a 45° angle to the pelvis; a non-slip seat surface with firm base is recommended
Ward (1984)		when a laptray is provided, it should place the gleno-humeral joint in 20-30° of flexion, with 90° of elbow flexion and forearms resting comfortably on the tray					
Hacker (1982)	provide needed support which does not restrict visual fields or voluntary movements			90° angle usually appropriate	foot support which keeps knees and ankles at 90°		lapbelt secured at a 45° angle across the hips
Trefler et al (1978)	head in midline with limited contact across occiput; if needed, use a neck collar to maintain midline		should be maintained in midline and as close to perpendicular position as possible	hips flexed at least to 90°; abduction pommel used as needed to keep knees separated	foot support placed so as to promote approximately 90° angle at ankles, knees, and hips		lapbelt should be secured at 45° to the pelvis, to keep the pelvis back in the seat

TABLE 1 (continued)

	HEAD	UPPER LIMBS	TRUNK	HIPS	KNEES	ANKLES and FEET	MATERIALS
Carrington (1978)		forearms should be at an approximate angle of 90° to the upper arm; desk should be 1/2 – 1 inch higher than the child's elbows, to provide adequate stability and movement		buttocks should reach close to the back of the chair to obtain hip angle of 90°, thus providing adequate hip flexion	back of the knees should not touch the front of the seat when the seat depth is adequate and hips are positioned correctly	feet should be positioned firmly on the floor, creating a 90° angle between the foot and the leg	
Motloch (1977)	held vertical with no stimulation over the occiput; use of neck support or doughnut-type headrest is recommended	shoulders vertical in the sagittal plane, rounded in the transverse plane	lumbar spine should be rounded	hips flexed 10–30° from horizontal and abducted; minimal stimulation over the ischial tuberosities	knees should be flexed to 90°	ankles should be at 90°, with minimal stimulation over the plantar surfaces	heavy weave upholstery (e.g., Herculon) allows skin ventilation and avoids skin tissue trauma; vinyl seating should be used only for incontinent clients

using therapeutic seating or other positioning devices. In general, the aforementioned authors provided some generic guidelines which encourage clinicians to promote midline orientation of the entire body, with near vertical alignment of the head and trunk. Foot support was strongly recommended. All authors implied that clients should be given the least amount of support which preserves the desired postural alignment, yet avoids restricting desirable active movement patterns.[4,38]

CLINICAL IMPLEMENTATION OF THERAPEUTIC POSITIONING

General Principles for Therapeutic Positioning

To determine the positioning needs for clients using alternative communication devices, an interdisciplinary team of clinicians should be employed. (See Attermeier, this issue, for discussion of interdisciplinary team process.) The combined expertise of the physical, occupational, and speech/communication-disorders therapists is essential in this process. Additional consultation by the physician, social worker, nurse, psychologist, educator, and equipment-vendor or engineer is often needed. In *no* case should consultation with the client's caretaker(s) be overlooked. For clients requiring complex interfacing of power wheelchair and electronic communication devices, the biomedical or rehabilitation engineer may be invaluable for assessment and execution of customized modifications.

Team members should be well-versed in the current spectrum of features, requirements, and disadvantages of specific communication units and positioning devices. Ideally, such components should be available for trial assessment with individual clients.

Positioning the client with significant musculoskeletal deformities, and fulfilling his or her need for an augmentative communication device is a challenge for the clinical team. McGee addressed this issue and summarized the myriad of problems facing the interdisciplinary team:

> The client, his family, and any involved medical and educational professionals may expect the seat to provide an optimal functioning position that gives good access to the environment to carry over therapy goals, to prevent or minimize abnormal muscle tone and abnormal movement patterns. If the client is totally dependent, the caretakers want a seat that is easy to use, maneuver, and keep clean. The client and his family are often concerned about the appearance of the seat, while the funding source is concerned with the cost. Often the needs expressed by this diverse group of individuals may differ.[38(p77)]

To attempt to meet the needs and expectations of the client and the individuals involved in his or her routine care, pre-planning for augment ative communication team evaluations is critical. In terms of efficiency, the team should anticipate those clinical specialties which will be needed for a given client. By having the client's caretakers and school or work personnel complete questionnaires prior to the assessment, many potential evaluation components may be identified. Pre-arrangements may be made with a neighboring facility or equipment vendor, to borrow an appropriate device or have an equipment representative available with a mock-up system suited to the client's anticipated needs. At the time of the planning meeting, consideration should be given to the home and school or work environment, architectural accessibility, and available transportation mode(s). For example, while the clinicians may be anticipating that a given client would be an ideal candidate for a power wheelchair interfaced with an electronic communication unit, the environmental assessment may reveal this to be an inappropriate recommendation because the client's home or family car cannot accommodate the power wheelchair.

Timing of the positioning intervention may also require considerati on; if the client is a candidate for corrective orthopedic surgery, it may be more judicious to postpone the selection of the seating system until the post-surgical period. Changes in skeletal alignment after surgery may influence the choice and need for specific adaptations for a positioning-communication system. Similarly, for clients who already have definitive seating-communication systems and later undergo corrective surgery, re-evaluation may be indicated to define re-adjustments for their systems.

Limitations of funding sources should be identified as early as possible, especially for clients having complex equipment needs. Alternate sources may be investigated by center-based or community-based personnel involved in the client's care. Designation of a community-based advocate is often desirable in this regard.

Incorporating Augmentative Communication with Therapeutic Positioning

With specific reference to clients using augmentative communication devices, Hacker stated that body positioning was important for: providing an upright posture for communication; facilitating educational input; improving the position of the lungs and diaphragm to allow better breath control and possibly better sound production; providing better orientation in space and improving spatial feedback; and improving upper extremity use by providing proximal stability.[3] Wilson also commented on the importance of integrating good body positioning for clients using oral or augmentative communication systems. She stated:

> Many children with cerebral palsy need to be upright to have enough breath support for speech. Children who use direct selection communication systems will need very carefully selected trunk and head supports in order to use their motor function for expression. Prone standers, corner chairs, and specially adapted wheelchairs or other modified chairs may be used to provide the support needed to promote communication skills. The therapist may find that a child needs more external control for tasks like communication but during times which are less stressful or less demanding on posture, the support can be removed so that the child uses the postural control that he is developing.[4(p173)]

Since an augmentative or alternative communication device must be accessed by some physical mode, evaluation of the client's neuro-musculo skeletal capabilities is essential. Schurman stated that the greatest percentage of children who need to use a communication board are non-ambulatory and, consequently, sitting position of the child in his wheelchair should be evaluated first. She added that in order to effectively indicate word choice on a communication board, the child must be able to maintain good posture throughout the day. For the child using a head-stick-pointing method, sitting posture was deemed even more important.[2]

Trefler and Taylor advised that each client's communication capabilities should be determined prior to the selection or prescription of the therapeutic seating system.[8] When the communication system is to be placed on the client's wheelchair tray or lapboard, the dimensions and position of the device must be carefully determined in order to maximize the client's ability to reach the individual communication units (e.g., pictures, symbols, or words on an electronic board), and yet permit convenient access to the switch or compatible unit needed to activate the device.

Trefler and Taylor also stated that these components are determined more accurately when the client is placed in a mock-up or simulated seating system.[8] Clinical adjustments of the simulator allows the staff to discover the limitations and advantages of their recommendations, and to permit an opportunity for problem-solving. The optimal components can then be replicated in the definitive seating system. Given the high cost of therapeutic seating and communication devices, simulation and problem-solving is essential to minimize the expense of potential errors in selecting the seating components.

An extended trial period with a mock-up system is critical for those clients who require integration of an augmentative communication unit with a power drive wheelchair. Placement of the control unit for the wheelchair must be established very carefully, via team consultation among the physical, occupational, and communicative disorders therapists. As a group, they must determine the most functional placement for the power drive unit, while minimizing loss of space and maintaining access to the communication unit. In many cases, the access device for the power wheelchair and the communication unit(s) will differ (e.g., use of a joy-stick control for wheelchair drive, with client accessing a word-board via head-stick pointer), requiring the therapists to develop creative strategies which the client can use to bridge these discrepancies. For example, use of overlays or thematic pages of pictures, words, or phrases can be used to maximize communication function with a minimum space requirement on a wheelchair tray. This type of problem-solving is very time consuming, often requiring several or more days of intensive evaluation and adaptation for a variety of situations which the client may encounter. For practical purposes, this assessment may be more efficiently administered during a short in-patient admission to the facility which specializes in such services. Once the evaluation has been completed, the appropriate equipment can be ordered and a readmission can be scheduled to fit the client with his or her customized system, providing training and additional problem-solving as needed.

The selected augmentative communication device must be adaptable to all of the positions in which the client is placed throughout the day. For individuals who are placed in a prone or supine stander, over a foam wedge or bolster, or in other positioning devices, the communication system must be accessible. Consultation and training with school or work staff, family members, or other caretakers should enable the clinical specialists to identify these needs and provide recommendations for incorporating the communication system into such alternative situations for each client.

SUMMARY

Positioning individuals with complex physical needs requires careful attention to many factors. An interdisciplinary team of experienced clinicians should be employed in this process, whenever possible. The team's duty is to incorporate the concerns and needs of the client's caretakers and community-based advocates and professionals, when the definitive system of positioning and communication is selected.

The existing literature on this subject matter is greatly in need of augmentation. Formal studies of the relationship between therapeutic positioning and functional use of augmentative communication devices have not been reported. Verification of the proclaimed purposes for using therapeutic positioning is also necessary. By taking *reliable*, serial goniometric measurements of passive joint ranges, clinicians would be better able to state that therapeutic positioning does indeed maintain joint motion and prevent contractures. Review of serial x-rays would also permit clinicians to determine if the application of carefully-selected therapeutic seating systems could minimize or actually prevent further deformities in those clients already being followed for mild to moderate scoliosis, hip subluxation, and other common orthopedic problems. Studies of functional capabilities before and after provision of an optimal positioning-communication system should also be repeated. This information could be easily retrieved during routine clinic visits or via written questionnaire or telephone survey administered to the client or caretakers.

Clinicians who work in settings where many clients are seen for positioning-communication devices have access to much of the data which is needed to document the effectiveness of our services in this specialty area. Although single-case presentations are often helpful in conveying creative solutions for positioning individual subjects, more formal studies of disability-specific populations seem to be in order.

Therapists are encouraged to consider biomechanical principles and related areas such as ergonomics, as they apply to muscle loading and endurance, energy consumption, and deforming forces which can alter structural alignment and function. The factors of endurance and fatigue are especially important for clients who require alternative communication modes: use of a head-stick pointer requires accuracy and finemotor control, but were the neck muscles designed to perform in this manner? What are the consequences of the compensatory neck and trunk movements over time? In this case, should we provide additional support to adjacent body parts (e.g., shoulders and trunk) in order to minimize neck muscular fatigue or compensatory re-alignment of the cervical vertebrae?

As technology advances, we will be required to keep pace in our assessment methods as well as our intervention approaches. Now is the time to augment our own defense of the proven benefits of therapeutic positioning for physically-handicapped individuals.

NOTES

1. Klein SD: New voices: Communication through technology. *Exceptional Parent* 13(3): 18-25, 1983.

2. Schurman JA: Custom designing communication board frames: The role of the occupational therapist, in Vicker BA (ed): *Non-Oral Communication System Project 1964/1973, University of Iowa Hospital School*. Iowa City, IA, Campus Publishers, University of Iowa, 1974, pp. 179-211.

3. Hacker B: The communication connection: Augmentative communication for the preschooler, in McLaurin S (ed): *The Preschool Special Child: Early Identification, Assessment and Management*. Chapel Hill, NC, Division of Physical Therapy, University of North Carolina at Chapel Hill, 1982, pp 162-170.

4. Wilson JM: Selection and use of adaptive equipment for preschool children, in McLaurin S (ed): *The Preschool Special Child: Early Identification, Assessment and Management*. Chapel Hill, NC, Division of Physical Therapy, University of North Carolina at Chapel Hill, 1982, pp 171-185.

5. Bergen AF, Colangelo C: *Positioning the Client with Central Nervous System Deficits: The Wheelchair and Other Adapted Equipment*. Valhalla, NY, Valhalla Rehabilitation Publications, Ltd, 1982.

6. Ward DE: *Positioning the Handicapped Child for Function: A Guide to Evaluate and Pre-*

scribe Equipment for the Child with Central Nervous System Dysfunction. St. Louis, MO, Phoenix Press, Inc, 1984.

7. Christopher RP: Medical indications and benefits of seating systems for children with cerebral palsy, in Trefler E (ed): *Seating for Children with Cerebral Palsy: A Resource Manual*. Memphis, TN, University of Tennessee Center for the Health Sciences, Rehabilitation Engineering Program, 1984, pp 25-31.

8. Trefler E, Taylor S: Decision making guidelines for seating and positioning children with cerebral palsy, in Trefler E (ed): *Seating for Children with Cerebral Palsy: A Resource Manual*. Memphis, TN, University of Tennessee Center for the Health Sciences, Rehabilitation Engineering Program, 1984, pp 55-76.

9. Wilson JM: Cerebral palsy, in Campbell SK (ed): *Pediatric Neurologic Physical Therapy: Clinics in Physical Therapy*, vol. 5. New York, Churchill Livingstone, 1984, pp 353-413.

10. Bleck EE: Severe orthopedic disability in childhood: Solutions provided by rehabilitation engineering. *Orthop Clin N Am* 9(2): 509-528, 1978.

11. Motloch WM: Seating and positioning for the physically impaired. *Orthot Prosthet* 31(2): 11-21, 1977.

12. Mital MA, Belkin SC, Sullivan MA: An approach to head, neck and trunk stabilization and control in cerebral palsy by use of the Milwaukee brace. *Dev Med Child Neurol* 18: 198-203, 1976.

13. Rang M, Douglas G, Bennet G, Kareska J: Seating for children with cerebral palsy. *J Pediatr Orthop* 1: 279-287, 1981.

14. Hulme JB, Gallacher K, Hulme, RD: The Montana adaptive equipment project: A cost-efficient model for the delivery of adaptive equipment services in rural settings. *Phys Occup Ther Pediatr* 1(4): 59-68, 1981.

15. Hulme JB, Schulein M, Hulme RD, et al.: Perceived behavioral changes in multihandicapped individuals using adapted equipment. *Phys Occup Ther Pediatr* 3(3): 63-73, 1983.

16. Trefler E, Nickey J, Hobson DA: Technology in the education of multiply-handicapped children. *Am J Occup Ther* 37(6): 381-387, 1983.

17. O'Brien M, Tsurumi K: The effect of two body positions on head righting in severely disabled individuals with cerebral palsy. *Am J Occup Ther* 37(10): 673-680, 1983.

18. Lee JM, Mahler TJ, Westling DL: Reducing occurrences of an asymmetrical tonic neck reflex. *Am J Mental Defic* 89(6): 617-621, 1985.

19. Nwaobi O, Smith PD: Effect of adaptive seating on pulmonary function in children with cerebral palsy. Rehabilitation Engineering Program, University of Tennessee, Memphis, TN 58163. Abstract of paper presented at National Conference of the American Physical Therapy Association, Chicago, June 1986.

20. Nwaobi OM, Brubaker CE, Cusick B, Sussman MD: Electromyographic investigation of extensor activity in cerebral palsied children in different seating positions. *Dev Med Child Neurol* 25(2): 175-183, 1983.

21. Nwaobi OM, Cusick B: The effect of hip flexion angle on the electrical activity of the hip adductors in cerebral palsied children (Unpublished report), 1980.

22. Heinrich MJ: Materials and fabrication techniques, in Trefler E (ed): *Seating for Children with Cerebral Palsy: A Resource Manual*, Memphis, TN, University of Tennessee Center for the Health Sciences, Rehabilitation Engineering Program, 1984, pp. 132-157.

23. Moore S, Bergman JS, Edwards G, et al.: The DESEMO customized seating support: Custom molded seating for severely disabled persons. *Phys Ther* 62(4): 460-463, 1982.

24. Carlson M, Winter R: The "Gillette" sitting support orthosis. *Orthot Prosthet* 32(4): 35-45, 1978.

25. Physical therapists making news: A profile of Carole Hunter. *Foundation for Physical Therapy NEWSBRIEFS*, Alexandria VA, September 1985.

26. Soderberg GL: *Kinesiology: Application to Pathological Motion*. Baltimore, Williams & Wilkins, 1986, pp 337-356.

27. Lattimore J, Stephens TE, Favell JE, Risley T: Increasing direct care staff compliance to individualized physical therapy body positioning prescriptions: Prescriptive checklists. *Ment Retard* 22(2): 79-84, 1984.

28. Nwaobi O: Biomechanics of seating, in Trefler E (ed): *Seating for Children with Cerebral Palsy: A Resource Manual*. Memphis, TN, University of Tennessee Center for the Health Sciences, Rehabilitation Engineering Program, 1984, pp 37-54.

29. LeVeau BF: Williams and Lissner: *Biomechanics of Human Motion*, ed 2. Philadelphia, WB Saunders Co, 1977.

30. Kapandji IA: *The Physiology of the Joints: The Trunk and the Vertebral Column, ed 2.* New York, Churchill Livingstone, 1974, p. 80.

31. Grieve GP: *Common Vertebral Joint Problems.* New York, Churchill Livingstone, 1981.

32. Ogden JA: *Skeletal Injury in the Child.* Philadelphia, WB Saunders Co, 1982.

33. LeVeau BF, Bernhardt DB: Developmental biomechanics: Effect of forces on the growth, development, and maintenance of the human body. *Phys Ther* 64(12): 1874-1882, 1984.

34. Norkin CC, Levangie PK: *Joint Structure and Function: A Comprehensive Analysis.* Philadelphia, FA Davis Co, 1983.

35. Bohannon R, Gajdosik RL, LeVeau BF: Relationship of pelvic and thigh motions during unilateral and bilateral hip flexion. *Phys Ther* 65(10): 1501-1504, 1985.

36. Carrington EG: A seating position for a cerebral-palsied child. *Am J Occup Ther* 32(3): 179-181, 1978.

37. Trefler E, Hanks S, Huggins P, et al.: A modular seating system for cerebral-palsied children. *Dev Med Child Neurol* 20: 199-204, 1978.

38. McGee M: Considerations in addressing the technical needs of the severely involved and/or institutionalized clients with cerebral palsy, in Trefler E (ed): *Seating for Children with Cerebral Palsy: A Resource Manual.* Memphis, TN, University of Tennessee Center for the Health Sciences, Rehabilitation Engineering Program, 1984, pp. 77-86.

Motor Assessment for Unaided and Aided Augmentative Communication

Shelley Stowers
Mary Ruth Altheide
Victoria Shea

SUMMARY. An appropriate match between the individual's motor skills and the motoric requirements of the augmentative communication system is a major factor in the selection of the system, therefore a thorough evaluation of motor abilities is a critical component of the overall evaluation. The primary components of a motor assessment and possible methods for obtaining this information are described. The major "unaided" or sign/gesture systems and their motor requirements are reviewed. Motor assessment for selection of an "aided" system requires identification of a mode of indication and range of indication, which are described herein. The three means of identification in aided systems (direct selection, scanning, encoding) and the motor skills they require are discussed. The therapist must integrate findings of the motor assessment with knowledge of the individual's communication needs and potential in order to select the most useful and complete system.

Selection of an augmentative communication system requires consideration of multiple factors (see Attermeier this issue). One major component that must be addressed is the individual's motor abilities, as motor output is an essential link between the individual and the chosen system. It is therefore vital for the interdisciplinary team to include a therapist with educational background and experience in normal and abnormal motor patterns (e.g., occupational or physical therapist). Coppola's[1] survey of occupational therapists involved in augmentative communication evaluations found that they were most frequently assessing physical status (motor abilities, somatosensory status, visual perceptual skills,) volition (motivation, occupational roles), and the environmental settings. One of the primary roles of the therapist involved in augmentative communication evaluations was the assessment of the individual's motor abilities in relationship to unaided and aided communication systems.

Shelly Stowers, MPH, OTR/L, Clinical Center for the Study of Development and Learning, CDL–BSRC 220H, University of North Carolina, Chapel Hill, NC 27514.

Unaided communication refers to techniques that utilize body parts and movements, usually the arms and hands (e.g., gestures and sign systems). Unaided communication can be either the primary mode or a supplemental technique of an augmentative communication system. Aided communication refers to techniques that utilize a physical object or device (e.g., manual board, electronic device). Current practice in the selection of an augmentative communication system emphasizes use of several augmentative techniques with a given individual to provide a means of communication in as many settings as possible, with and without equipment. Such a system may include an electronic device, a manual board, and a gesture/sign system.

The purpose of this article is to provide the therapist with information on the primary components of motor assessments for unaided and aided augmentative communication. As each individual's communication needs and motor abilities are different, no universal format for motor assessments has been developed. No established criteria for selecting the most appropriate motor response mode are available. Information from the motor assessment must be integrated with the therapist's knowledge of normal and abnormal motor patterns and available communication techniques, as well as with the contributions of other team members.

SCREENING

Initial evaluation of voluntary motor patterns and active range of motion of the upper extremities can serve as a screening mechanism to indicate whether an unaided, aided, or combination system would be most appropriate. The therapist must have knowledge of the individual's cognitive abilities and communication needs and potential, as decisions must be made regarding whether the motor system can support the unaided or aided communication needs. Areas for consideration during this motor screening include: (1) the ability to maintain postural and head control during movement, (2) the variety and quality of available movements, (3) the ability to isolate one joint movement from another, (4) the effect of voluntary movement on associated movements throughout the body, (5) reflexes and involuntary movements, and (6) contractures and deformities. Based on this information, a decision about proceeding with a thorough unaided or aided motor assessment can be made. Because unaided systems require refined motor skills, they can often be ruled out as a primary mode of communication for individuals with severe motor impairments. In that case, the therapist should proceed to the aided motor assessment, as information regarding available movements for a supplemental unaided technique (e.g., reliable yes/no response – eyes look up for yes, head shake for no) can be gained through this evaluation procedure.

UNAIDED MOTOR ASSESSMENT

One of the essential steps in matching an individual with a sign or gesture system involves consideration of the individual's motor ability compared with the motor requirements necessary to produce the sign or gesture. The relationship of sign characteristics to sign acquisition and retention has gained recognition in the past decade,[2] however, the relationship of the motor abilities of potential sign users to the motoric components involved in sign production has been addressed by very few authors. Many individuals have been selected to use signs with little or no information available on the individual's motoric competencies.[3,4] Dennis and associates[5] cited studies which indicated that over 10,000 persons in the special needs population were involved in sign programs but that motor skill requirements were seldom considered when selecting signs.

Systems exist for analyzing the components of individual signs. Commonly used terms for sign differentiation are: (1) designator (dez) – the configuration of the hand, (2) tabula (tab) – the location of the sign relative to the body, (3) signation (sig) – the movement or action of the hands, and (4) orientation (or) – the orientation or plane of the palm of the hand.[6] Doherty[2] simplified these categories to handshape, location, movement and orientation. Multiple specific motor components exist within these categories: voluntary movement patterns, active range of motion, unilateral and bilateral movement patterns, motor planning abilities and sequential motor movements.

Models for Motor Assessment

Dunn[7] and Dennis and associates[5] used a developmental motor model as a foundation for an unaided motor evaluation. Dunn[7] identified three characteristics of signs as important factors in analyzing motor components: (1) the relationship of the sign to the body (movement of the sign toward or away from the body, face or midline), (2) hand use patterns (unilateral and bilateral movement, dominant/assister control and reciprocal movements patterns), and (3) hand shapes (position of fingers). Dunn also identified the factors of movement combined with touch and movement performed within the visual field as important variables. Following developmental analysis, Dunn[7] suggested that signs optimal for imitation: (1) have movement toward the body; (2) are performed at or toward, but not across midline; (3) are performed with touch; (4) are within the signer's visual field; and (5) are performed with the forearm in neutral or pronated position. Similarly, Dennis and associates[5] identified three motoric factors to be considered in sign selection: (1) prehension movement patterns, (2) unilateral/bilateral movement patterns and (3) combination of successive actions. The influences of motor planning, tactile contact, and visibility of the movement pattern were also addressed by this author. These authors have provided excellent resources describing motor skill assessment for unaided communication.

Methods of Motor Assessment

The unaided motor assessment can include both formal and informal procedures. Information on motor behaviors can be gathered through: (1) observing an individual interacting with toys or materials, (2) engaging in activities of daily living, (3) administering motor assessment tools (to provide clinical information as it relates to signs) and (4) administering motor imitation tasks. Although motor patterns are often assessed through imitation tasks, Dennis and associates[5] report two problems associated with this method: (1) poor imitators may not provide reliable information regarding which motor patterns are available to them and (2) some individuals who do not perform the movement patterns in isolation may be able to perform them in the context of other motor movements. Therefore, it is often advantageous to use more than one method to gather information on motor behaviors.

Content of Motor Assessment

Active Range of Motion and Voluntary Movement Patterns

This area was addressed initially in the screening process. If the decision was made to administer a thorough unaided motor assessment, additional information on an individual's upper extremity movements and range of motion is necessary. Voluntary, involuntary, and associated movement patterns and the inability to execute specific movement patterns require documentation. More important, while screening provided information on gross movements, more assessment of refined movement and prehension patterns is needed. Evaluation of the individual's ability to isolate fingers and sustain finger patterns necessary for sign formation provides the therapist with information about the individual's ability to produce specific handshapes. The dominant hand warrants particular attention because of the skill requirement of most sign systems. Dennis and associates[5] provide charts which analyze prehension movement patterns, the sign alphabet and activities of daily living as they relate to sign production.

A number of assessment tools are available to assist the therapist in gathering motor information. The choice of tools depends on the individual's cognitive abilities and level of physical impairment. Dennis and associates[5] reported that the tools most commonly used in assessing fine motor skills for unaided communication were: the S.E.E.D. Fine Motor Developmental Profile,[8] Fine Motor Developmental Test[9] and Prehension Assessment.[10] The Fine Motor subscale of the Peabody Developmental Motor Scales[11] or any other comprehensive fine motor developmental test can also be used.

Unilateral/Bilateral Movement Patterns

The ability of the individual to produce unilateral upper extremity movements will have been well documented from the assessment procedure described above. Bilateral patterns of dominant/assister, simultaneous, and reciprocal movements now require assessment. Dennis and associates[5] identified seven specific developmental categories of unilateral/bilateral movement patterns necessary for sign production: unilateral not across midline, bilateral mirror movements, bilateral movements, unilateral across midline, bilateral one base-one mover, bilateral both movers, and bilateral crossing midline with two hands. Several assessment tools are available to gain clinical information on the child's use of these movements. Dennis and associates[5] suggest the following commonly used assessment tools: the Purdue Perceptual Motor Survey—Imitation of Movement Subtest,[12] Meeting Street School Screening Test,[13] and the Motor Accuracy, Imitation of Postures, Kinesthesia and Tactile Perception and Space Visualization subtests of the Southern California Sensory Integration Tests.[14] The new but not yet available Sensory Integration and Praxis Tests[15] includes promising subtests of Bilateral Motor Coordination, Postural Praxis, Sequencing Motor Praxis and Praxis on Verbal Command. The Imitation of Gestures Test[16] is also useful.

Motor Planning and Sequencing of Motor Movements

Motor planning is defined as the ability to plan and smoothly execute a motor task. Because signing is a dynamic process, planning of the motor movements and specific handshapes directly involve motor planning abilities. Speed and accuracy of sign production is also related to motor planning skills. A sign may require different beginning/ending handshapes or a sequence of motor actions (compound signs). Fluid production of more than one sign (word) utterance requires a sequence of motor responses. The number of successful motor sequences a child can produce provides information about the ability of the motor system to support the length of utterance needed to express complex thoughts. The assessment tools listed in the unilateral/bilateral section are also helpful in assessing this area.

UNAIDED COMMUNICATION SYSTEMS

Numerous gestural and sign systems are used around the world. Gestures lack linguistic structure and tend to be transparent, i.e., having a clearly understandable meaning based on form alone. Although transparency is an advantage, the backgrounds and experiences of the user and message receiver must be similar in order for correct message interpretation to occur. Sign systems, however, are languages that follow individual patterns of grammar and syntax. As long as both the user and receiver know the language, they can communicate even though their backgrounds may be very different. Sign languages are capable of conveying much more complex information than are gestural systems.

Selection of an unaided system requires knowledge of the variety of options and their characteristics. Musselwhite and St. Louis[17] compared features of nine gestural communication systems: American Sign Language, Signed English, Signing Exact English, Duffy's System, Fingerspelling, Cued Speech, Amer-Ind, Natural Gestures and Pantomime. Features they chose for comparison were cognitive demands, interpretation, linguistic structure, vocabulary size and motor requirements. The motor requirements of each system were classified into three categories: gross, moderate or fine movement. In addition, primary use of either one or two hands was specified. Of the nine gestural systems compared, four required primarily fine motor control (American Sign Language, Signed English, Signing Exact English, and Fingerspelling), two required moderate control (Cued Speech and Amer-Ind), and three required only gross control (Duffy System, Natural Gestures, and Pantomime). With the exception of two systems (Fingerspelling and Cued Speech), all required use of two hands. Therapists should be familiar with the following systems, as they represent the major sources of gestures and signs in use with non-vocal individuals.

American Sign Language

The unaided system most widely used by the deaf in the United States and Canada is American Sign Language (ASL)[18] or Ameslan. ASL is a language in and of itself, not a code to represent English or any other language. This language has capabilities for simultaneous coding of several pieces of linguistic information, which makes it an efficient technique. ASL combines manual signs with nonmanual signals of facial expression, body orientation and eye gaze. Musselwhite and St. Louis[17] indicate that candidates for use of ASL should demonstrate good motor control of both hands in order to produce the 19 basic hand configurations. Signs in ASL are produced at a variety of places relative to the body and with a number of movement patterns, therefore, good range of motion in both arms is a factor.

Although ASL was developed as a communication system for the deaf, its successful use has been reported with other populations such as the mildly to profoundly mentally retarded[19-21] and other non-vocal individuals who are multihandicapped.[22,23] In many cases the clients using ASL demonstrated success with isolated signs (lexical entries) or with two and three sign strings rather than with ASL as a total system. ASL signs tend not to be transparent in nature, thus limiting the audience of message receivers. Klima and Bellugi[24] found that of 90 ASL signs presented to subjects who knew no signs, 81 signs were not guessed. They also found that signs were not readily transparent even when presented in a multiple choice fashion.

Shane and Wilbur[25] have established a procedure for predicting the ability of a given motor-impaired individual to use ASL signs. They began by analyzing the motor requisites in the production of signs. Categories of location, handshape and motion were computer analyzed to determine the motor requisites using a vocabulary of 2,637 ASL signs from *Dictionary of American Sign Language* (DASL). The analysis revealed the following breakdown: (1) location – chest area 44.9%, hand 27.8%, and face 22.2%; (2) hand shape – flat hand shape 38.8%, isolated index finger 28.5%, fist 15.2%, curved hand 10.9% and thumb touch 5.4%; (3) motion – linear 56.6% and rotate/twist 11.1%. Movement occurred in 87.5% of the DASL entries. These authors advocated the comparison of motor control of the individual with the motor skills necessary to produce intelligible signs.

In a small descriptive study, Diener[26] analyzed motor aspects of 158 commonly used ASL signs. She reviewed more specific components than those used by Shane and Wilbur[25] choosing instead categories to represent the broad developmental stages as proposed by Dunn.[7] This description may provide the therapist with more specific information regarding the motor abilities needed by the signer and the necessary modifications required in establishing a vocabulary. For example, of the 158 commonly used ASL signs, 41% required forearm supination; if an individual were unable to supinate, significant modifications would be necessary or a decision made as to whether the use of the signing system as a primary technique for communication was viable. Diener found 61% of the signs to be combined with touch and 63% to be combined with vision. Forearm placement during sign production was reported to be 53% with forearm pronated, 41% with supination and only 8% with the forearm in neutral. Thirty-seven percent of the ASL signs involved unilateral movement and

22% bilateral hand movement. Of the 158 signs, 23% involved dominant assister patterns and 16% reciprocal patterns. Whole hand signs were involved in 56% of the ASL signs, with isolation of finger groups necessary for 43%. Six percent of the signs analyzed required sequential movement to produce an individual sign.

Signed English

While based in part on ASL, Signed English [27] varies in content and form. Signed English was originally designed for the hearing impaired preschool population, and provides a structured approach for learning English through signs. Signs follow English syntax and are produced in the same order as the spoken language. More than 3,000 signs are available in the current system. Fourteen sign markers allow for addition of grammatical features (e.g., plurals and tense). Words and word forms that are not covered by the vocabulary are formed through fingerspelling, a code which uses 26 distinct handshapes to represent the 26 letters of the Roman alphabet. The motor control required for use of Signed English is equivalent to that needed for ASL. If fingerspelling is included, more discrete control is required.

Amer-Ind Gestural Code

This code is based on Universal American Indian Hand Talk. The system was modified by Skelley and Schinsky[28] to include 250 clinically tested signals (signs) covering concepts expressed by the 1000 most frequently used English words. No grammatical structure is used with the signals. Concepts are conveyed by means of hand position and movement sequences to allow for expansion or specificity. There is no one correct signal for an idea; specific interpretation is determined by the context. Transparency of Amer-Ind was initially reported by Skelley and Schinsky[28] to be 80-90%. More recent research shows Amer-Ind to be approximately 50% guessable for non-retarded young adults.[29-31] Exclusive of the number signals, the clinical repertoire contains 236 signals. Of these, 131 are normally executed by one hand (either left or right). Of the remaining 105 signals, 94 can easily be adapted for one hand execution.

Duffy's Innovative Sign System

Duffysigns is a system developed for the physically handicapped.[32] The 471 signs are formed by gross motor gestures and are combined with vocalizations. Gross volitional control of all limbs is necessary to use this system. Some signs require use of two hands or active use of legs. Moderate control of facial musculature is necessary, as many signs involve use of lips or facial expression. This output system allows for execution of letters, numbers, and single or combined signs. Duffy created this system for use within a closed environment, thus assuring that the message receiver would be familiar with the system. Typically Duffysigns are used to communicate basic information, however options for extended messages using combined signs or spelling exist.

AIDED MOTOR ASSESSMENT

The primary purposes of the motor assessment for aided communication are the identification of a *mode* of indication and documentation of the *range* of indication. This provides information for selection of a *means* of indication.

A mode of indication is the method an individual uses to access a communication device. The mode may be a voluntary motor response (e.g., finger pointing), or a voluntary motor response used in conjunction with a switch or adaptive equipment (e.g., head movement and headpointer). The voluntary movement selected for a mode of indication should be the most accurate, efficient, reliable and readable movement available to the individual. Identification of such a movement is often difficult for individuals with severely limited voluntary movements, and may therefore require extensive assessment. Once the most controlled voluntary movement is identified, adaptive equipment and modifications can sometimes be included to make it more accurate and readable.

The range of indication is the physical space which the mode of indication can accurately and consistently reach. For example, an individual's range of indication may be limited to several inches on either side of the midline of the body.

The means of indication is the way in which the mode of indication interacts with the communication device to relay the individual's message. Three basic approaches are available for providing an individual with a means of indication: direct selection, scanning and encoding. The mode of indication directly interacts with the means of indication.

Direct selection is defined as any technique in which the desired choice is directly indicated by the user.[33] Examples of a direct selection mode are pointing a finger or looking at an object or picture. Direct selection is the fastest, most direct way of responding, and of the three means of indication requires the least cognitive ability. If at all possible, a direct selection mode of indication should be identified, because of its speed and easy readability.

Scanning is defined as any technique in which an array of selections is offered to the individual by a person or device and the individual signals when the desired choice is presented.[33] The individual may signal with a yes/no response or with a switch that has been connected to a device. The mode of indication for scanning can be a single voluntary motor response. If a switch and electronic device are used however, controlled response timing is essential. A significant disadvantage of scanning is the slow rate of communication, since many selections may need to be offered before the individual's choice appears. Numerous scanning techniques exist, however, some of which can increase the speed of communication.[17] Three examples of scanning techniques are linear, row/column and directed.

The slowest form of scanning, linear, involves choices presented one at a time with the individual responding when the desired choice is located. In row/column scanning, rows are presented sequentially; when the row containing the desired item is reached, the individual activates the switch in order for scanning to begin within that row. The switch must again be activated when the location of the desired choice is found. Directed scanning may employ a single switch (e.g., joystick) or multiple switches (e.g., armslot control switch) which the individual directs to the desired location. This is one of the fastest scanning processes, but can require greater motor control than the linear and row/column scanning methods.

Encoding is defined as any technique in which the desired choice is indicated by use of a code (e.g., Morse Code). Multiple encoding possibilities exist, such as coding by color or number. For example, for an individual with poor motor accuracy, a color code system could be employed by putting two words within each location on a communication board. Each word would have a different color background (e.g., white and yellow); the individual would indicate a selection by first choosing the color and then the desired location. For an individual with limited range of indication, but extensive vocabulary needs, a number encoding system could be utilized. Number encoding could involve numbering each word, and having the individual select specific numbers corresponding to desired words. Encoding requires good cognitive and memory skills, and can be coupled with direct selection and scanning. When integrated with direct selection, encoding can increase the amount of available vocabulary for individuals with limited accuracy and range of indication. When used with scanning, encoding can provide faster access to vocabulary, and therefore increased rate of communication. Multiple resources are available to assist therapists in designing encoding systems.[17,33-35]

An individual should not be limited to only one mode of indication if his or her motor and cognitive abilities will support more than one, since each mode of indication allows access to different augmentative communication techniques. An individual needing a complete augmentative communication system will find it useful to have multiple options for mode of indication, and each individual should have at least one direct selection mode of indication. Early introduction of the use of headpointers and light beam indicators is recommended.

Methods of Motor Assessment

Many assessment formats are available for determining the most appropriate mode of indication (see resource list). Forms developed by the Augmentative Communication Program at the Clinical Center for the Study of Development and Learning[36] for the documentation and dissemination of information relating to an individual's augmentative communication system are located in the Appendices. A survey of occupational therapists involved in motor assessment for aided communication revealed that informal evaluations using center-developed formats were the most frequently used methods for making decisions about the mode of indication. Trial and error formats were reported as most frequently used for switch and electronic device decisions.[1] No established criteria exist for identification of the most appropriate mode of indication as each nonvocal individual presents unique motor skills, cognitive abilities and communication needs. The therapist must usually gather information through informal procedures and make decisions based on clinical information.

General Motor Considerations

The initial step in an aided motor assessment is providing the individual with optimal positioning (see Mac Neela this issue). Once the individual is positioned, the voluntary movements are assessed. The therapist must be aware of the effect that voluntary movement has on associated and involuntary movements, reflexes, and contractures or deformities. Voluntary movements often elicit associated and involuntary movement which can interfere with accuracy and response time, and encourage contractures or deformities.

The initial screening process described in this article addressed the assessment of voluntary movement patterns and range of motion of the upper extremities. If the decision was made to administer a thorough aided motor assessment, the following additional components require evaluation. They will be addressed according to the means of indication categories and presented in a format reflecting a suggested progression.

Direct Selection

The suggested progression of assessment in this category is: hand and fingers, head, and eye movements. The primary components of this assessment process are:

Range and Accuracy of Movement. Initially the range of indication for functional, controlled movement must be investigated. Additional analysis of motor accuracy or "resolution" must occur in order to establish the cell size which will allow for interpretation of a clear, readable response. Coleman, Cook and Meyers[37] described resolution of motion as the minimal movement which a client can reliably and accurately execute. Use of grids with various cell sizes to determine range and accuracy of movement is suggested. Goossens and Crain[38] provided additional information on determining the optimal response mode. The goal of their procedure is to determine a direct selection response mode which will allow for the largest range of motion to accurately target the smallest cell size within the least amount of time. This procedure involves use of selected modes of indication (e.g., finger, manual pointer, headpointer, light beam indicator) and a variety of laminated grids containing different cell sizes. The clinician records range, accuracy in targeting cells, time required to locate cells and overflow movements associated with responding throughout the trials. When determining range and accuracy of movement the therapist should be careful not to require a cognitive response while assessing motor abilities. For example, the therapist should not require an individual to point to an orange triangle if he or she is uncertain of the individual's color and shape recognition skills.

Activation Techniques. The individual's ability to sustain and release specific movement and to exert pressure requires evaluation. This becomes an issue when an electronic device or switch is being considered. Electronic devices and switches vary in their activation techniques. Some require sustained movement (e.g., optical viewpoint indicator) while others require pressure for activation. Evaluation of an individual's ability to produce, sustain and release pressure is important, as too little pressure may not activate the device, whereas too much pressure may activate multiple repetitions of the intended response. Evaluation for determining activation techniques, therefore, is most easily accomplished by specific device and switch trials.

Response Time. The amount of time an individual requires to initiate and release a movement has a direct impact on the speed of communication. This factor should be considered when evaluating the best response mode. For example, an individual may be a faster responder with a head light than when using his or her upper extremities. This issue of response time is important when considering a switch-operated scanning system, as most systems have a limited response time available.

Repetition of Response. The ability of an individual to repeat a response is an important factor, because augmentative communication requires multiple repetitions. For some individuals, the effects of a repeated response may be increased fatigue and decreased accuracy or speed.

The factors of range and accuracy of movement, activation techniques, response time, and repetition of response should be evaluated when considering a manual pointer, headpointer, mouthpointer, or use of a light beam indicator. Use of keyguards, angle of materials (e.g., 30 degrees from table top) and placement of materials (e.g., right of midline) are other variables which the therapist should consider as these can have significant impact on motor performance.

Eye Movements

The use of eye gaze as a mode of indication requires special assessment. The individual's ability to fix, track and scan should be evaluated, as should the ability to maintain an eye gaze accurately enough to be read by the receiver. This can be accomplished using a plexiglass sheet, approximately 24″ × 30″ with a central quadrant (5″ × 6″) cut out. The individual looks at the therapist through the cut out quadrant, and then at various locations on the plexiglass sheet. Use of pictures or stickers at various locations, or simply having the therapist point to different locations will provide information on the readability of the response. The therapist should note the individual's ability to maintain head control and to isolate eye movements from head movement. Locations of accurate eye gaze and the range of indication of eye gaze should be documented (see A & B in Appendix I). Numerous eye gaze communication systems are available.[17,33,38] Once the individual's eye gaze abilities and cognitive/communication needs are documented, an appropriate eye gaze system can be chosen.

Scanning

For the severely motorically involved individual, use of a switch connected to a device may be the only available mode of indication for communication. Switches can also be used to access battery operated toys, environmental controls, call signals and computers, as well as provide independent mobility (e.g., power wheelchairs). When assessing for switch use, identification of at least one voluntary motor response is necessary, as commercial or customized switches are available to match most voluntary movement patterns (e.g., tread switch, mercury switch, joystick, latching switch). The suggested progression of assessment for control sites is hand/fingers, upper extremities, and head, although any body part, including foot or knee, demonstrating consistent control could be considered. Once a voluntary movement is identified, trials with switches that activate battery-operated toys or a tape recorder may assist the therapist in assessing the factors of activation pressure, response time, repetition of response, and type and positioning of the switch.

More systematic assessments for single input switches are available. The single input control assessment was developed by the Ontario Crippled Children's Center and described by Goossens and Crain.[35] This procedure for evaluating alternate control sites was developed for use with the physically handicapped. Two components are involved: (1) clinical: designed to determine three options for single input control and (2) computer assisted: designed to evaluate systematically and objectively the individual's performance using the three options selected in the clinical portion. During clinical trials, information is gathered relating to four components (MSIPs): M-movement pattern, S-control site, I-switch interface, P-positioning of switch.

The Control Evaluator Training Kit (CETK)[39] developed by The Children's Hospital at Stanford is an additional tool for systematic, quantitative assessment and training for use of controls with assistive devices. This system outlines three major steps in selection of a control (1) site selection, (2) control selection and (3) comparative testing of control site and control combinations. Controls which can be used with the CETK include: single switches, switch arrays, joysticks and small keyboards.

Encoding

Encoding is a strategy for accommodating motor limitations to provide increased accessibility of vocabulary. Motor components requiring evaluation have been previously discussed.

Device Characteristics

Selection of the optimal response mode will provide information relating to communication device options. Specific device characteristics may solve some of the problems which occur with an individual presenting motor limitations. Some specific devices may be ruled out as the individual may not demonstrate the motor ability needed to activate the device. The following discussion is not meant to reflect individual characteristics of specific devices, but to reflect device characteristics which can affect the mode of indication. Familiarity with device characteristics, motor information, and the considerations discussed by Attermeier in this issue will assist the therapist in the client/device match.

Manual Devices

Manual devices (e.g., manual communication boards) tend to allow for greater customization than do electronic devices. When fabricating a communication board, range of indication and accuracy of movement can be adjusted to meet an individual's motor abilities. Displays may have uniform cells (all 1″ × 2″) or variable cell size (left of midline 1″

squares/right of midline 2″ squares). Goossens and Crain[35] proposed a method to customize communication displays of variable cell size. Vocabulary can be placed within the individual's range and encoding strategies can easily be included (see C in Appendix I).

Electronic Devices

Electronic devices can provide an individual with specialized qualities such as voice output, written output, and memory components. The therapist must match the selected mode of indication characteristics (e.g., range, accuracy of movement) with the device access characteristics. For example, electronic devices may be accessed through pressure membrane switches, light emitting diodes or keyboards for direct selection. Some devices can be regulated to accommodate a range of activation forces. Other devices can be regulated to accommodate different activation times (i.e., amount of time needed to remain on a location). A variety of electronic devices can accommodate a variety of scanning systems and many include a delay feature which allows for accommodation of an individual's reaction time (see D in Appendix I).

SUMMARY

While multiple factors must be considered in determining the viability of an unaided communication system, one major component that must be addressed is the individual's motor abilities. Information was provided on the primary components of a motor assessment, as were possible methods for conducting the assessment. Descriptions of various sign systems and their motor requirements were reviewed.

The primary purposes of the motor assessment for aided communication are identification of a mode of indication and documentation of the range of indication. The three basic approaches relating to the means of indication and their interaction with the mode of indication were discussed. Information was provided on the primary components of a motor assessment and adaptive equipment options. Descriptions of various device characteristics which affect motor ability were reviewed. This information will assist the therapist in determining an appropriate motoric match between the individual and the device.

NOTES

1. Coppola S: *Current Practice of Occupational Therapists in Augmentative Communication*, thesis. University of North Carolina at Chapel Hill, Chapel Hill, NC, 1985.

2. Doherty J: The effects of sign characteristics on sign acquisition and retention: An integrative review of the literature. *Augment Altern Commun* 1:108-121, 1985.

3. Goodman L, Starks-Wilson P, Bornstein H: Results of a national survey of sign language problems in special education. *Ment Retard* 16:104-106, 1978.

4. Reichle J, Williams W, Ryan S: Selecting signs for the formulation of an augmentative communicative modality. *J Assoc Sev Hand* 6(1):48-56, 1981.

5. Dennis R, Reichle J, Williams W, et al.: Motoric factors influencing the selection of vocabulary for sign production programs. *TASH Journal* 7:20-31, 1982.

6. Stokoe W: *Sign Language Structure*. Silver Spring, MD, Linstok Press, 1978.

7. Dunn M: *Pre-Sign Language Motor Skills*. Tucson, AZ, Communication Skill Builders, 1982.

8. Herst J, Wolfe S. Jargansen G, et al.: *S.E.E.D. Fine Motor Profile*. Tacoma, WA, Sewall Early Education Development Program, 1976.

9. Montgomery P, Richter E: *Sensory Integration for Developmentally Disabled Children: A Handbook*. Los Angeles, CA, Western Psychological Services, 1978.

10. Holstein R: *Prehension Assessment*. Madison, WI, Waisman Center on Mental Retardation and Human Development, 1980.

11. Folio MR, Fewell R: *Peabody Developmental Motor Scales and Activity Cards*. Allen, TX, DLM Teaching Resources, 1983.

12. Roach E, Kephart N: *Purdue Perceptual Motor Survey*. New York, Charles E. Merrill, 1966.

13. Hainsworth P., Sequeland M: *Meeting Street School Screening Test*. Providence, RI, Crippled Children and Adults of Rhode Island, 1969.

14. Ayres AJ: *Southern California Tests of Sensory Integration*. Los Angeles, Western Psychological Services, 1966.

15. Ayres AJ: *Sensory Integration and Praxis Tests*. Los Angeles, Western Psychological Services, in press.

16. Berges J, Lezine I: The imitation of gestures. *Clinics in Developmental Medicine No. 18*, London, England, The Spastics Society Medical Education and Information Unit in Association with William Heinemann Medical Books Ltd, 1965.

17. Musselwhite C, St. Louis K: *Communication Programming for the Severely Handicapped: Vocal and Non-Vocal Strategies*. Houston, TX, College-Hill Press, 1982.

18. Stokoe W, Casterline D, Croneberg C: *Dictionary of American Sign Language* (rev. ed.) Silver Spring, MD, Linstock Press, 1978.

19. Hobson PA, Duncan PD: Sign learning and profoundly retarded people. *Ment Retard* 17:33-37, 1979.

20. Simpson MA, McDade HL: A Total Communication Approach in an Interdisciplinary Infant Development Program. A paper presented at the American Speech-Language-Hearing Association Convention, Atlanta, GA, 1979.

21. Stremel-Campbell K, Cantrell D, Halle J: Manual signing as a language system and as a speech initiator for the nonverbal severely handicapped student, in Sontag E (ed): *Educational Programming for the Severely and Profoundly Handicapped*. Reston, VA, Council for Exceptional Children, Division on Mental Retardation, 1977, pp 335-347.

22. Koselka MJ, Hannah EP, Gardner JO, et al.: Total Communication Therapy for a Non-Deaf Child and his Family. A paper presented at the American Speech and Hearing Association Convention, Washington, DC, 1975.

23. Konstantareas MM, Oxman J, Webster CD: Iconicity: Effects on the acquisition of sign language by autistic and other dysfunctional children, in Siple P (ed): *Understanding Language Through Sign Language Research*. New York, Academic Press, 1978, pp 213-237.

24. Klima ES, Bellugi U: *The Signs of Language*. Cambridge, MA, Harvard University Press, 1979.

25. Shane H, Wilbur R: Potential for expressive signing based on motor control. *Sign Lang Stud* 29:331-48, 1980.

26. Diener P: Motoric Aspects of Signs, unpublished paper, Clinical Center for the Study of Development and Learning, University of North Carolina, Chapel Hill, NC, 1985.

27. Bornstein H, Saulnier KL, Hamilton LD: *The Comprehensive Signed English Dictionary*. Washington, DC, Gallaudet College Press, 1983.

28. Skelly M, Schinsky L: *Amer-Ind Gestural Code Based on Universal American Indian Hand Talk*. New York, Elsevier Publishing Company, Inc, 1979.

29. Doherty J, Daniloff J, Lloyd L: The effect of categorical presentation on Amer-Ind transparency. *Augment Altern Commun* 1:10-16, 1985.

30. Doherty JE, Karlan GR, Lloyd L: Establishing the transparency of two gestural systems by mentally retarded adults. *ASHA* 24:834, 1982.

31. Imhoff TE, McMillen MH: The transparency of Amer-Ind and S.E.E. to untrained peers. *ASHA* 26:10, 1984.

32. Duffy L: *An Innovative Approach to the Development of Communication Skills for the Severely Speech Handicapped Cerebral Palsied Children*, thesis. University of Nevada, Las Vegas, NV, 1977.

33. Vanderheiden G: Providing the child with a means to indicate, in Vanderheiden G, Grilley K (eds): *Non-Vocal Communication Techniques and Aids for the Severely Physically Handicapped*. Austin, TX, Pro-Ed, 1977, pp 20-76.

34. Silverman F: *Communication for the Speechless*. Englewood Cliffs, NJ, Prentice-Hall, Inc, 1980.

35. Goossens C, Crain S: *Augmentative Communication Assessment Resource*. Lake Zurich, IL, Don Johnston Developmental Equipment Inc, 1986.

36. Altheide MR, Stowers S, Porter P, et al.: Augmentative Communication Forms, Clinical Center for the Study of Development and Learning, University of North Carolina, Chapel Hill, NC, 1985.

37. Coleman C, Cook A, Meyers L: Assessing non-oral clients for assistive communication devices. *J Speech Hear Disord* 45:515-526, 1980.

38. Goossens C, Crain S: Eye-Gaze Communication Systems: Assessment and Intervention. A paper presented at Fifth Annual Southeast Nonspeech Communication Conference, Birmingham, AL, 1984.

39. Barker M, Hastings W, Flanagan K: The Control Evaluator and Training Kit: An Assessment Tool for Comparative Testing of Controls to Operate Assistive Devices. A paper presented at the Sixth Annual Conference on Rehabilitation Engineering, San Diego, CA, 1983.

AIDED MOTOR ASSESSMENT RESOURCE LIST

A Resource Manual for the Development and Evaluation of Special Programs for Exceptional Students
Vol. III-M
Procedures for an Interdisciplinary Evaluation of Nonoral Students
FDLRS Clearinghouse/Information Center
Bureau of Education for Exceptional Students
Division of Public Schools
Florida Department of Education
Knott Building
Tallahassee, FL 32301

Assistive Devices Center Assessment Forms
California State University at Sacramento
600 J Street
Sacramento, CA 95819

Augmentative Communication Assessment Resource
Carol Goossens and Sharon Crain
Sparks Center for Development and Learning Disorders
University of Alabama in Birmingham
1720 Seventh Avenue, South
Birmingham, AL 35233

Augmentative Communication Evaluation Form
Pacific Northwest Non-Vocal Communication Group
Children's Orthopedic Hospital
University of Washington Hospital
Seattle, WA

Augmentative Communication Evaluation and Questionnaire for Home and School
Clinical Center for the Study of Development and Learning
(Division for Disorders of Development and Learning)
University of North Carolina at Chapel Hill
BSRC 220 H
Chapel Hill, NC 27514

Credit Valley Treatment Center for Children
Assistive Devices Resources Program
2277 South Millway
Mississauga, Ontario L5L 2M5
Canada

Pre-Verbal Communication Schedule
Assessment of Pre-Communicative and Non-Verbal Communicative Behaviour
Chris Kiernan
Thomas Coram Research Unit
University of London Institute of Education
41 Brunswick Square
London WC1N 1AZ, England

Augmentative Communication: Selection of an Initial Vocabulary

Patricia B. Porter

SUMMARY. Selection of an initial vocabulary is a critical element in the implementation of any augmentative communication technique. This article reviews the literature on the subject then proposes a procedure to be used in selecting vocabulary for aided techniques. Content guidelines, selection strategies and vocabulary expansion methods are delineated.

Selection of an initial vocabulary is a critical element in the assessment and implementation of an augmentative communication technique; the user will find little motivation in the use of a sophisticated technique if the vocabulary does not facilitate functional communication. While an augmentative communication user will overcome great physical obstacles, inappropriately prescribed devices and poorly designed interfaces to access a useful vocabulary, the opposite situation does not occur.

The purposes of this article are (1) to review information on selection of an initial lexicon, and (2) to delineate a comprehensive set of strategies for vocabulary selection for the nonspeaking person who has never used language functionally.

LITERATURE REVIEW

One of the earliest elaborations on the importance of selecting a vocabulary was made by Vanderheiden and Harris-Vanderheiden in 1976.[1] They listed a set of basic considerations and directed that the vocabulary system chosen should:

1. be compatible with the aid or technique with which it will be used;
2. place the least amount of restriction on the child's communication;
3. be appropriate to the child's current expressive ability;

Patricia B. Porter, PhD, CCC-Sp, Assistant Professor, Speech and Hearing Services and Director of Clinical Programs, Clinical Center for the Study of Development and Learning, CDL-BSRC 220H, University of North Carolina, Chapel Hill, NC 27514.

4. be developmental and flexible in order to allow for the child's changing communication needs;
5. be adaptable to current therapy and educational procedures and approaches; and
6. be acceptable to the child, his parents and teachers and those with whom he will communicate.

Elder and Bergman[2] described a procedure in which children were taught to identify Blissymbols by directed eye gaze. They noted that the selection of particular symbols was determined by the environment and needs of the individual. No information was presented regarding functional use of the symbols trained via this protocol.

Nietupski and Hamre-Nietupski[3] described a two step process for initial vocabulary selection. The first step involved generating a pool of possible items using student preference, frequency of occurrence, functional utility across situations and basic human needs. The second step involved refining the list by selecting topically dissimilar vocabulary symbols. Significantly, Nietupski and Hamre-Nietupski[3] identified student motivation as a major factor in system use. They note that "It would seem reasonable that if a student has a favorite toy, food, activity or person, the instructor can arrange a situation in which the student is taught to communicate in order to obtain the favorite objects, activities or persons."[3(p118)]

Selection of a core vocabulary to be used with Bliss or Rebus symbols was the focus of a paper by Wilson.[4] She felt that the lexicon should involve the consideration of the individual, his environment, the characteristics of the specific system and normal language acquisition. The lexicon selection process, Wilson suggested, should involve a variety of people including parents, teachers and the individual himself.

A format for individualizing vocabulary selection was presented by Carlson[5] in 1981. She proposed a child-centered, situationally oriented vocabulary based on the work of McDonald and Schultz[6] and Vicker.[7] Teachers, parents, clinicians and others, as well as the child, provided input on the selection. She noted a need for such a format in that some children "failed to develop any symbolic communication with a preselected lexicon."[5(p241)] Initially, the cause for this failure was thought to be inappropriate device or symbol system selection but when the vocabulary was modified, the children began to use the system appropriately. Carlson proposed a format for the vocabulary pool which incorporated a parent interview form and the identification of the child's environmental settings. The child's ability to interact in these settings was evaluated by making site visits to sample areas. The speech/language pathologist then presented categories of words and asked the adult in each of the settings to find all the words appropriate to that setting which fell into that category. For instance, the teacher might select the following words for the "activities" category: puzzles, book, swing, outside. The speech/language pathologist then constructed an initial vocabulary by selecting from these lists words which were at or below the child's developmental level and were of interest to the child.

A behavioral-remedial strategy for vocabulary selection based on developmental considerations was demonstrated by Karlan and Lloyd.[8] This involved inventory of the individual's environments and student preferences, frequency of occurrence and functional utility of potential items and basic human needs. The authors noted that because preferences change, frequent re-evaluation is necessary. In addition, they suggest that "routine opportunity to choose between several options will increase the need to communicate during activities associated with the fulfillment of human needs."[8(p14)] Karlan and Lloyd presented sample vocabulary lists for elementary and adolescent aged severely handicapped people and they presented social validation data to determine the usefulness of each. This validation procedure employed judges who had contact with one of the two age groups. The authors pointed out that these samples were not the only vocabularies possible and that particular preferences of the user could well replace other items.

None of these studies advance any data on the actual efficacy of the vocabulary selection strategies on the functional use of augmentative communication systems. Much additional study is needed in this area both for mechanical systems as reviewed here and also for electronic and gestural communication systems.

PROPOSED CONTENT GUIDELINES FOR A FIRST VOCABULARY

Bearing in mind that the goal is functional communication, the first symbols selected to be displayed on an augmentative communication device must be functional, reinforcing, reinforceable, and not already present in the user's communicative repertoire.

Functional

Yoder and Kraat[9] suggest that "strict adherence to a vocal communication development and use model may not be appropriate for the population, if effective communication is our goal."[9(p29)] While color labels may be well within the developmental boundaries for a particular child, it is doubtful that the use of such labels would prove immediately functional. Rather, those words or phrases which serve to solve the user's most frustrating communication problems (e.g., "more" or "hurt") would be far more functional.

Reinforcing

Communication must allow the user to employ, at first, symbols representing his or her personal preferences. Motivation is a critical factor and a first vocabulary with items truly reinforcing to the *user* motivates him or her to use the system. Care should be taken not to impose words reinforcing to the message receiver among these first items. "Bathroom," while very useful to a primary caretaker may not be particularly reinforcing as a first item for the non-toilet-trained child.

Reinforceable

Functional communication is a powerful event because it allows the individual to have tremendous impact on the environment. As 10- to 12-month-old infants begin to utter their first meaningful words, they quickly learn that utterance of the word "cookie" frequently produces a cookie and that "mama" garners gleeful attention (not to mention the repeated echo of the word). This same power must be an integral part of the use of the first vocabulary. The first words selected, therefore, must be immediately reinforceable by presentation of that object, activity or person as a consequence for the user's selection of it. A picture of a roller coaster may be tremendously reinforcing and appropriate to add to a display prior to an amusement park visit. It is not, however, appropriate as a first lexicon item because the system user will not be able to immediately experience the consequence of his or her choice.

The immediate receipt of the choice is a critical component of this step. Eventually, once the use of the technique is learned, immediate consequences are less critical, and one can then respond to the system user in much the same way one responds to a speaking person. A request for a snack may be met with the reply "I see that you want a snack, John. It's not quite time, but you can have one in twenty minutes."

Items Not *Present in Current Communicative Repertoire*

Traditional learning theory directs that to teach a new skill, the instructor begins at the point of a student's highest competency level related to the new task and then teaches the new task relying on that known skill as a basis. This would lead us then, to an understanding that the best first vocabulary for an augmentative system would be those "words" already spoken or gestured by the new system user. Unfortunately, this theory does not translate well into the development of communication. If the system user already has a way to successfully communicate a "word," placement of the "word" on the system display as a first vocabulary item only serves to provide a communicative hurdle for the system user. Why should he now use this system to communicate something which he is able to communicate already, often more rapidly. The system should solve rather than create communicative problems. Eventually objects, persons, activities and feelings represented by semi-intelligible speech or personal gesture can be placed on the display so that all message receivers can understand. The first vocabulary, however, must include items about which the user has no current means to communicate.

PROPOSED SELECTION STRATEGY

Within content guidelines, vocabulary items can be selected in a number of ways. Functional words can best be identified by observing the system user in his multiple communicative environments. What does he need to say in the home, sheltered workshop, group home or classroom? An abundance of information can be gathered by observing the communication of his peers and particularly by observing those unsuccessful communication situations in which the system user is most frustrated. Words which often emerge are those reflecting feelings, past or future events or very specific items. Others in the user's environment can also be helpful in adding to this list.

Knowledge of the system user's preferences is essential. Porter and colleagues[10] have described a systematic procedure for identification of preferences. The procedure includes lists of potentially reinforcing objects and activities and means to evaluate responses which indicate pleasure or displeasure. This is sometimes not easy when the young woman with cerebral palsy has a smile that at times looks like a grimace. The identification of preferences is critical as items are selected which are reinforcing and reinforceable.

Observation and interview provide the best information on the system user's current communication. The therapist should observe the individual in all communicative environments and interview those persons who act as primary message receivers. Be cautious only to include those items which are fairly consistently identified as having certain meaning to familiar listeners. When in doubt, you can often verify the intent of a word or gesture by checking with the system user.

VOCABULARY EXPANSION

Initial vocabulary items should be placed on the display in such a way that vocabulary can be easily expanded. The goal, in most instances, will be grammatically correct, multiple word utterances. Placement toward this sort of expansion is illustrated in the Appendix.

The vocabulary needed will often exceed the system user's range and specificity of indication. Increase in vocabulary without increase in range or specificity can occur by employing multiple sequential displays,[7] which take the form of a flip chart (Figure 1). The first page can serve as a menu for subsequent pages which can be categorized and color coded. Multiple simultaneous displays[7] expand the vocabulary and facilitate correct use of grammar (Figure 2) since each list of words in a particular

FIGURE 1. Multiple Sequential Display (adapted for visual gaze)

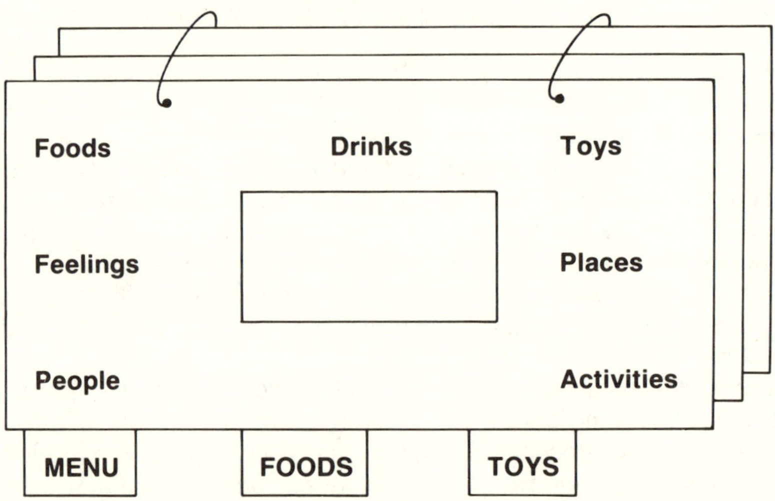

FIGURE 2. Multiple Simultaneous Display

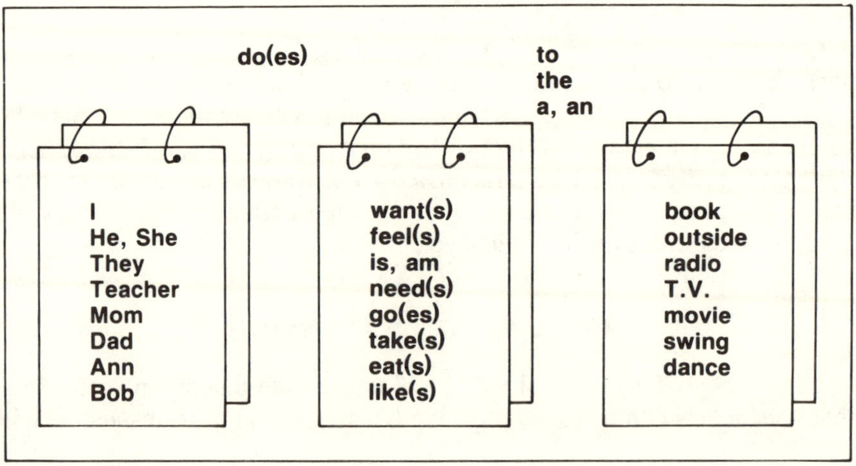

class can be independently accessed and displayed. Finally, the alternate word strategy can expand vocabulary without increasing indication specificity (Figure 3). Second words are added within the system user's most specific pointing area, and the words are color coded. The system user, when indicating the new word in that area, first indicates "I am selecting a red word" then he or she touches that area. The message receiver knows then that the color coded word in that segment is the one being selected.

For some system users, vocabulary needs will increase quite rapidly. Many strategies can be used to systematically expand the lexicon. Three frequently used strategies are listed here:

1. *Observed Need* – the system user has a tablet attached to his system at all times; when there are points of breakdown in communication, the word(s) when finally identified are written in the tablet. When the words appear twice within a week, they are included on the display.
2. *Systematic Categorization* – begin to categorize object nouns placing foods in one line, activities in a second and so on. These categories can be color cued for ease of visual identification.
3. *Specificity of Selection* – add modifiers so that instead of the "ball," the system user can now request the "big, red, ball."

SUMMARY

Selection of the initial vocabulary is an extremely important step toward the functional communicative use of an augmentative communica-

FIGURE 3. Alternative Word System

Bold Print = Red Word

do(es) not

the
a, an

I	want(s)	big	ball	tired
Ann	**Eat(s)**	**yellow**	**swing**	**hot**
He, She	Like(s)	sharp	puzzle	happy
Doug	**Drink(s)**	**green**	**dog**	**uncomfortable**
They	Feel(s)	pretty	pencil	angry
Erin	**Go(es)**	**orange**	**TV**	**caught**
Teacher	Need(s)	cold	doll	sick
Rachel	**Take(s)**	**purple**	**radio**	**wet**
Mom	See(s)	red	car	bad
Pat	**Have, Has**	**my**	**movie**	**furious**
Dad	am, is, am	blue	block	good
Rover	**Hear(s)**	**your**	**VCR**	**o.k.**

tion system. Literature in this area describes selection strategies but does not address the impact of these strategies on actual, functional communication. The suggestions in this article have been directed to use of mechanical, aided augmentative systems. Guidelines for selection of a first vocabulary and vocabulary expansion techniques have been described. Similar attention must be given to the development of strategies for both electronic aided systems and gestural communication systems.

REFERENCES

1. Vanderheiden G, Harris-Vanderheiden D: Communication techniques and aids for the nonvocal, severely handicapped, in Lloyd L (ed): *Communication Assessment and Intervention Strategies*. Baltimore, University Park Press, 1976.
2. Elder P, Bergman JS: Visual symbol communication instruction with nonverbal, multiply handicapped individuals. *Ment Retard* 16 (2): 107-112, 1973.
3. Nietupski J, Hamre-Nietupski S: Teaching auxiliary communication skills to severely handicapped students. *Am Assoc Educ Sev Prof Handicapped Review* 4 (2):107-124, 1979.
4. Wilson KD: Selection of a core lexicon for use with graphic communicative systems. *J Child Comm Disabil* 4 (2):111-123, 1980.
5. Carlson F: A format for selecting vocabulary for the nonspeaking child. *Lang Speech Hear Serv Schools* 12:240-245, 1981.
6. McDonald E, Schultz A: Communication boards for cerebral palsied children. *J Speech Hear Disabil* 38:73-88, 1973.
7. Vicker B: Advances in nonoral communication system programming: Project summary #2, in Vicker B (ed): *Nonoral Communication Project, 1964-1973*. Iowa City, IA, Campus Stores, 1974.
8. Karlan GR, Lloyd LL: Considerations in the planning of communication intervention: Selecting a lexicon. *J Assoc Sev Hand* 8:13-25, 1983.
9. Yoder D, Kraat A: Intervention issues in nonspeech communication, in Miller J, Yoder D, Schiefelbusch R (eds): *Contemporary Issues in Language Intervention ASHA Reports #12*. Rockville, MD, ASHA, 1983.
10. Porter PB, Carter S, Goolsby E, et al.: *Prerequisites to the Use of Augmentative Communication Systems*. Chapel Hill, NC, DDDL-BSRC, 1984.

APPENDIX

Progression of Placement of Vocabulary Selections on Mechanical Communication Devices for Correct Grammatical Sequence

I. Begin by placing first vocabulary selections (objects and activities) to the right of center. When the technique user responds functionally to these selections move to the next step (Figure 4).

II. Place *I want(s)* together on the left side of the board. Require the user to point to *I want(s)* then one of the objects or activities to make a complete selection (Figure 5).

III. Gradually separate *I* and *want(s)* placing *want(s)* in a category to the right of *I*. Require the user to touch *I want(s)* object/activity to get what he wants (Figure 6).

IV. The next step usually involves placing *He* and *She* under *I* and including several proper names (*Dad, Mom, Mrs. Jones*, etc.) (Figure 7).

V. Begin to gradually add objects and activities to that category. In most instances you will move from a generic "*food*" to kinds of foods and kinds of toys, etc. (Figure 8).

VI. Gradually increase the verbs to include *like, need, have*, etc. (Figure 8).

VII. Place *Do (does) not* at the top of the verb category (Figure 8).

VIII. Add a category for feelings to the right of the objects/activities (*hot, cold, tired, angry*, etc.). Be sure to add *feel(s)* to the verb category at the same time (Figure 9).

IX. Gradually add to each of the categories as necessary (Figure 9).

X. Add a category of auxiliary verbs to the left of the verb category (Figure 9).

XI. Add a category of modifiers to the left of the objects/activities category (*big, little, red, his, hers, theirs, more*, etc.) (Figure 9).

XII. Add *and, the, a*, to the top of the object/activity category. Add *-ed, -ing* and *to* to the top of the modifier category (Figure 9).

XIII. At this point, the user has the opportunity to indicate complete, grammatically correct sentences.

Cautions:

(1) If at any point the user seems frustrated, slow down and leave the vocabulary alone for several days.

(2) The strategy described above is a *training* strategy. No system user should be required to make grammatically correct utterances all the time. For most day to day social purposes a one word response is adequate. Use normal verbal communication as a guide.

FIGURE 4. Objects/Activities

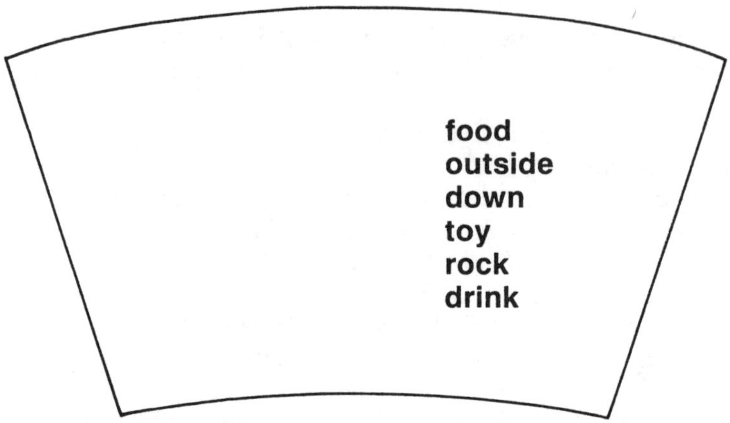

FIGURE 5. Two Step Request

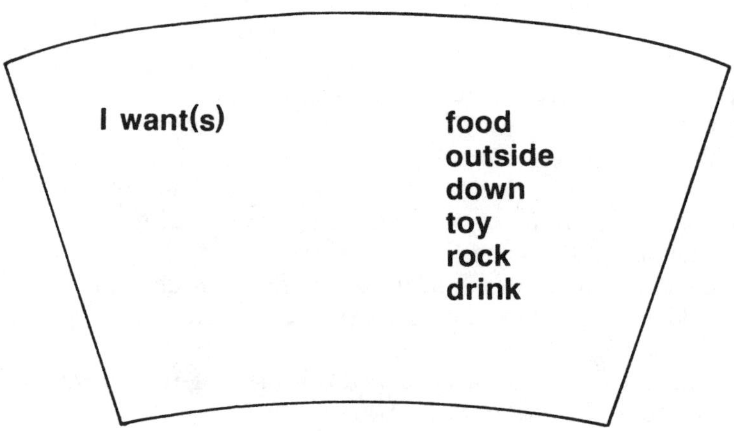

FIGURE 6. Three Step Request

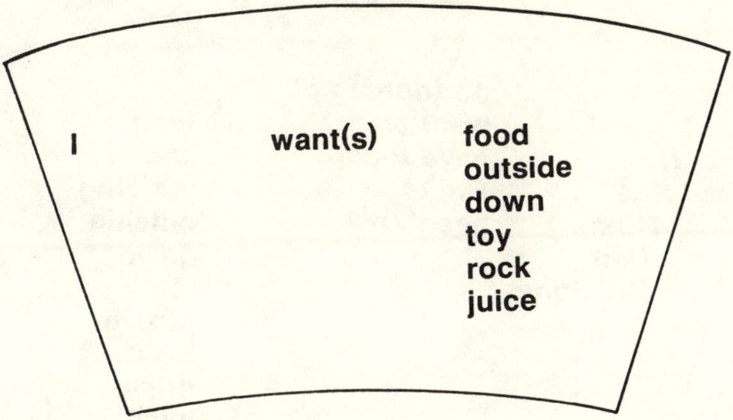

FIGURE 7. Expanded Subject List

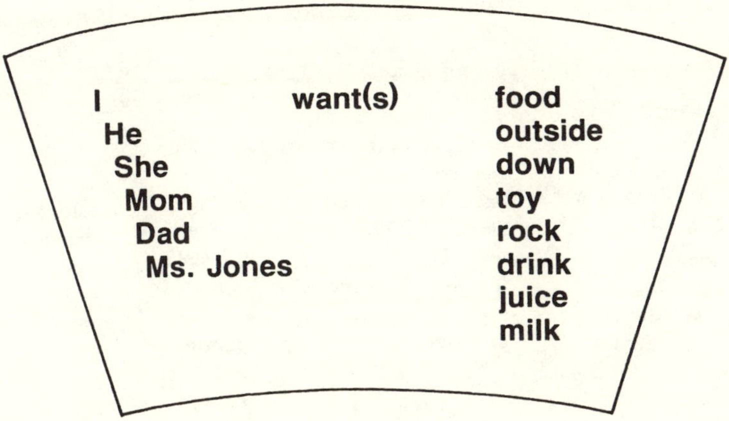

FIGURE 8. Expanded Verb and Object List

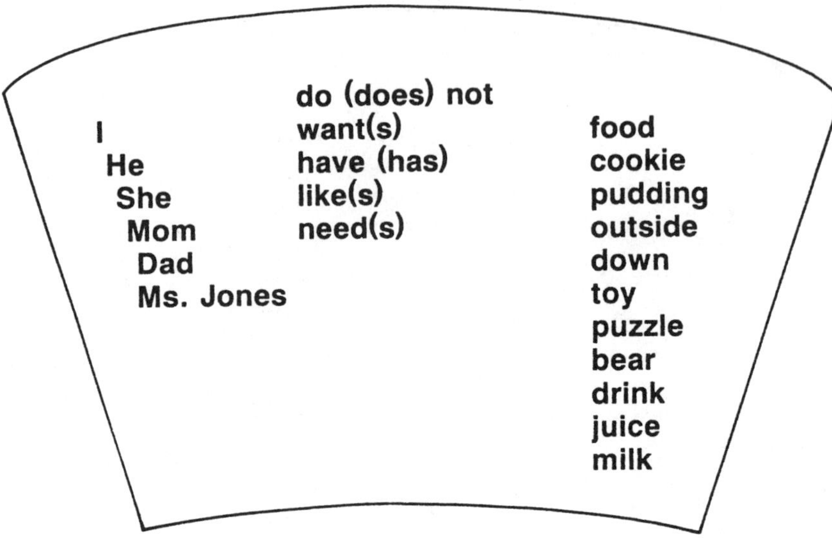

FIGURE 9. Modifiers and Feelings

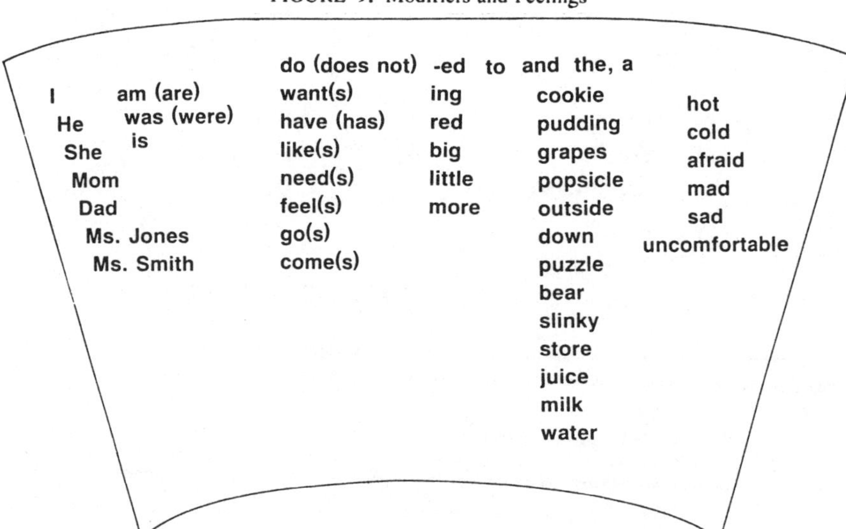

Language vs. Communication in Training for Augmentative Communication System Use

Patricia B. Porter

Provision of an augmentative communication system is not enough; training in the *use* of the system must follow. Yoder and Kraat[1] noted that "how we view the teaching/intervention process has been crucial to the user's success." Traditionally, receptive labeling has been the first step in language training.[2,3] The sequence of the program ordinarily proceeds by presentation of an object, picture or word accompanied by the cue "show me the ______." The therapist reinforces the child or adult's correct selection by saying "good" then moving on the next object, picture or word. A second option has been a shaping, modeling and differential reinforcement strategy proposed by Risley and Wolf,[4] Lovaas[5] and many others. While this sort of receptive vocabulary training continues to have merit in some situations, it is not appropriate as the first step in augmentative communication training. First, Sleigh[6] has shown that a picture of one object, clearly represented, or a miniature object is not recognized by normally developing children until about 18 months of age. This is comparatively late to begin training the preliminaries to the use of an augmentative communication system. Second, no clear relationship exists between the ability to identify object, picture or word labels and the use of objects, pictures or words for functional communication. Yoder and Kraat[1] expressed the concern that many of our failures to teach appropriate system use may be due to "frequent preoccupation with form rather than interaction or communication."[1(p314)]

Augmentative communication training should, more appropriately, progress in much the same way as normal expressive language development. At nine months of age babies are able to make reliable choices between objects presented to them, even though they do not necessarily know the names of the objects. They then progress to functional use of the referents for these objects (usually spoken words) to control their environments. Goetz, Schuler, and Sailor[7] noted that abilities to concep-

Patricia B. Porter, PhD, CCC-Sp, Assistant Professor, Speech and Hearing Sciences and Director of Clinical Programs, Clinical Center for the Study of Development and Learning, CDL–BSRC 220H, University of North Carolina, Chapel Hill, NC 27514.

tualize tools to achieve desired environmental outcome are vitally important in early language development and enhance the development of early lexicons. Choice making is the first step. It precedes comprehension of "yes" and "no" questions (Early Stage v – 2-3 years) in the developmental sequence. Potential augmentative communication system users need not know the names of words, pictures or objects for training to proceed. Training should begin with choice making and proceed in normal developmental sequence for expressive language.

Review of the literature reveals that various training strategies have been used to initiate the use of augmentative communication systems with nonspeaking children and adults. These strategies fall into two major categories: (1) language training – direct teaching of receptive and expressive word labels and grammatic structure and (2) communication training – indirect training of the use of objects, pictures or words for functional expression of information. In some studies training represents combinations of these strategies.

Murdock[8] described a training program with a fifteen-year-old mentally retarded girl. Traditional speech therapy using shaping, modeling and differential reinforcement had been employed and, after eleven years, the young woman had use of only one spoken word. Murdock[8] used a multiple baseline technique to evaluate the effects of training the young woman to identify written words on request. She found that differential reinforcement by saying "good" or "that's right" increased rate of responding on the two words and two phrases to a rate of 90-100% accuracy. Murdock reports that after this training the young woman was using the word cards to "communicate in the classroom."[8(p24)] No description of this communication or follow-up study were reported.

Nietupski and Hamre-Nietupski[9] proposed a process to teach auxiliary communication skills to severely handicapped students. The program employed physical assistance, imitation, prompting and maximum teacher intervention to encourage independent performance by the student. They also proposed that these auxiliary skills be employed twenty four hours a day across instructional activities with strong parental support using a concurrent skill cluster orientation with comprehension and production being trained simultaneously.

Yoder[10] proposed teaching/intervention strategies which crossed both persons and environments and included: (1) early social stimulation, (2) reinforcing early intentions, (3) teaching language structure and form, (4) demonstrating effective use of nonverbal behavior, and (5) emphasis on communicative functions and use.

Porter and colleagues[11] described a training protocol beginning with identification of preferences and establishing a reliable mode of response. The sequence then moves to use of this mode of response to make choices between two objects and gradually moves to reliable choice making among four pictured objects or activities. This provides the seed for the development of a functional communication system.

In his chapter on intervention strategies, Silverman[12] includes a list of general concepts. Among these, he lists generating motivation to communicate and increasing awareness of the nature of communication. He encourages giving the nonspeaking person opportunities to make decisions such that he or she can know the benefits of communication.

Dunst and Lowe[13] proposed a system of incidental teaching episodes which can be employed every time the child is in the presence of another person. These include steps to: (1) ensure child responsiveness to environment through opportunities that secure and maintain the child's attention, (2) focus attention on those aspects of the environment that maintain attention, (3) elicit and sustain the child's interactions with the environment, (4) work for and sustain elaboration in child's topography of behavior, and (5) work for and sustain conventionalization as part of response elaboration.

DISCUSSION

Culp and her colleagues[14] in a recent report of aid use in Texas noted a high percentage of aid rejection and low percentage of aid use. This trend has been reported before. Yoder and Kraat[1] noted that "it is very possible that poor use of augmentative systems and the reduced levels of communication . . . are directly connected to our current intervention goals and procedures."[1(p48)] Professionals must recognize that those who use augmentative communication systems may not benefit from traditional language therapy. Rather, training directed toward functional use of the system with all the inherent reinforcing qualities of expression built in, may lead to more effective system use. Finally, more data based research needs to be conducted comparing various training procedures.

NOTES

1. Yoder D, Kraat A: Intervention issues in nonspeech communication, in Miller J, Yoder D, Schiefelbush R (eds): *Contemporary Issues in Language Intervention: ASHA Reports 12*. Rockville MD, American Speech, Language, Hearing Association, 1983.

2. Van Riper C: *Speech Correction: Principles and Methods*. Englewood Cliffs, NJ, Prentice Hall, 1965.

3. Berry M, Eisenson J: *Speech Disorders: Principles and Practices of Therapy*. New York, Appleton, Century, Crofts, 1956.

4. Risley T, Wolf M: Establishing functional communication in echolatic children. *Behav Res Ther* 5:73-88, 1967.

5. Lovaas I; *Reinforcement Therapy* (16 mm film). Philadelphia: Smith, Kline and French Laboratories, 1966.

6. Sleigh G: A study of some symbolic processes in young children. *Brit J Comm Dis* 6:163-175, 1972.

7. Goetz L, Schuler A, Sailor W: Motivational considerations in teaching language to severely handicapped students, in Goetz L, Schuler A, Sailor W (eds): *Behavior Therapy for the Developmentally Disabled*. New York, Academic Press, 1983.

8. Murdock JY: A nonoral expressive communication program designed for a nonverbal retardate. *J Child Comm Dis* 2(1):18-25, 1978.

9. Nietupski J, Hamre-Nietupski S: Teaching auxiliary communication skills to severely handicapped students. *A AESPH Review* 4 (2):107-124, 1979.

10. Yoder D: Interaction strategies for augmentative communication use. Presentation to N.C. Augmentative Communication Association, Raleigh, NC, May 6, 1984.

11. Porter P, Carter S, Goolsby E, et al.: *Prerequisites to Augmentative Communication*. Chapel Hill, NC, Division for Disorders of Development and Learning, 1984.

12. Silverman F: *Communication for the Speechless*. Englewood Cliffs, NJ, Prentice-Hall, 1980.

13. Dunst C, Lowe LW: From reflex to symbol: Describing, explaining and fostering communicative competence. *AAC Augmentative and Alternative Communication* 2(1):11-18, 1986.

14. Culp D, Ambrosi DM, Berniger TM, Mitchell J: Augmentative communication aid use – a follow-up study. *AAC Augmentative and Alternative Communication* 2(1):19-24, 1986.

Supporting Families of Augmentative Communication Users

Mary Ruth Altheide
Jean R. Livermore

SUMMARY. As knowledge and understanding in the field of augmentative communication increases, professionals have become increasingly aware of the value of involving family members in developing, using and adapting an augmentative communication system. Parents bring different levels of knowledge and skills, as well as different feelings and levels of acceptance, to this process. Team members need to understand the strengths, stresses and needs of the family in order to work together effectively.

The time of initial evaluation and the recommendation for an augmentative communication system provides ideal opportunities for engaging families. Families need professional guidance, and professionals need family input to determine the most effective communication system for their clients. Parents often need assistance with the difficult and time-consuming process of locating funding for equipment purchase. Moreover, once a working relationship is established, families will continue to rely on professionals in many areas. As clients' communication skills increase over time, systems will need adaptation and revision; therefore the relationship between families and professionals is ongoing. A cooperative effort supports both the client and the family, and contributes to the successful use of the augmentative communication system.

FAMILY INVOLVEMENT IN AUGMENTATIVE COMMUNICATION

The first major professional recognition of the need to involve families in the augmentative communication evaluation process occurred in 1980, in *Nonspeech Communication: A Position Statement* by the American Speech-Language-Hearing Association (ASHA).[1] In this document the client and family were identified as members of the interdisciplinary evaluation team, and consideration was given to their needs when determining appropriateness of an augmentative communication system. In

Mary Ruth Altheide, OTR/L, Clinical Center for the Study of Development and Learning, CDL – BSRC 220H, University of North Carolina, Chapel Hill, NC 27514.

addition, ASHA identified the need to disseminate information to professionals, parents, and nonspeaking persons.

The importance of the perspective of parents of handicapped children and their participation in program planning and implementation continues to be recognized.[2] In 1980, Montgomery[3] supported and defined the role of parents as members of the interdisciplinary assessment and training teams. Suggested parental roles included supplying input on communication needs in the home and community, commenting upon practical applications of the proposed system, supporting training team activities, using the system in the home when appropriate, and suggesting improvements for functional use of the communication system. Shane and Bashir[4] also acknowledged the importance of parents and other family members in the successful use of augmentative communication systems.

Klein[5] observed that as children gain experience with communication they become more actively involved with other people. Changes were noted at school and home; as the children's skills in expressing their thoughts improved, parents and teachers appeared to become more responsive to them. The children appeared happier as improved communication with friends and relatives was possible. This is understandable, since human relationships are based on communicative interaction. Moreover, the primary relationships are within the family. The family remains the basic unit by which we care for, nurture, support, teach and socialize our children. We do this through communication. Parents know this intuitively, as they eagerly await the baby's first smiles, first vocalizations, and first words. The primary learning setting for communication is within the family—the most personal kind of interaction occurs here. Other social systems (school, church, agencies) may interact directly with the child, but as long as the child remains dependent on the family, the values, perceptions, attitudes and priorities of the family unit will be more important and have more "weight" than those of people outside the family. Professionals, therefore, must understand the nature of communication within the family if they are to devise a functional communication system. A communication system that is not appropriate for the family will not be accepted by it and will not be used in the home setting, thus denying the child the opportunity to utilize the system in the environment of primary human relationships. Augmentative communication systems are too costly to design, both in time and money, for professionals to risk other than maximum benefits for their clients.

In 1986 ASHA prepared an evaluation matrix to be used while improving the use of communication aids in schools serving handicapped children.[6] Parental involvement is identified as a critical component throughout the goals, objectives and criteria set forth in the matrix. Some of the strategies mentioned include: fostering active participation of the family, including the family as a part of the interdisciplinary team, facilitating use of a variety of augmentative approaches during family-directed activities, cooperation between home and school through daily or weekly written communication, and providing formal mechanisms for ongoing training regarding communication aids and interventions in order to enhance the augmentative communication user's interaction with family members. Active participation of the family and client on the interdisciplinary team during formation and update of the Individual Education Plan or Individual Program Plan, providing instruction in basic communication interaction processes for the family and soliciting feedback from the client's family about effectiveness of the program on a regular basis are also identified.

CLINICAL ISSUES WITH FAMILIES

Family Assessment

Once the utility of family involvement is accepted and areas where family participation would be beneficial are identified, the professionals need to develop strategies for maximizing family members' interest and investment in the process. These will differ for each family, as families will vary in the levels of interest, energy, and skills they are able to apply to the process. Thus, an initial and primary need is for a social/emotional assessment of the family. At the Clinical Center for the Study of Development and Learning, a clinical social worker is included on the Augmentative Communication Team. The social worker conducts family assessments, provides social information to other team members, and, along with other team members, maintains an ongoing relationship with the family. Family assessment provides information about family strengths that will support the continued growth and learning of the client, and family stress that may interfere. A major part of this assessment consists of determining the family's current ability to accept the client's handicaps, as this will have a major impact on their acceptance of a system.

Much has been written about parental response to the birth of a handicapped child. Many factors affect the family's ability to accept and adjust to this crisis including: (1) the degree to which the child differs from parental expectations; (2) family composition (birth order of child); (3) health and age of parents; (4) socio-economic status; (5) individual personality of parents and child; (6) stage in the family life cycle; (7) extent of the handicap and other characteristics of the child; (8) availability of outside support systems; and (9) religious and cultural values.[7]

As parents come to terms with the loss of the anticipated normal child, their response may follow a normal pattern of grieving that is recognizable and expected. Parents often have an initial period of disbelief (denial), and are likely to experience powerful feelings of anger, depression and guilt before coming to acceptance of the child's condition and their situation. Blacher[8] has reviewed the literature, and proposes that these feelings may not follow a predictable sequence but may exist at different times and with different intensities, based on factors such as the degree of the handicap and family characteristics. Thus the presence of these feelings at different times in the adjustment period is considered normal. They may be expected to last for some time period, and are only considered problematic if their duration or intensity is such that it prevents the parent from caring appropriately for the child or moving on with his or her own life. Moreover, the parent is likely to re-experience this grief over and over again, as life events bring reminders of the child's handicap—a phenomenon known as chronic sorrow.[9] Such grieving typically occurs at times of normal developmental milestones for the child—walking, talking, entering school, adolescence—as parents watch other children moving through these stages and are reminded of the contrast between those children and their own.[10]

Thus the lack of development of speech has particular impact in two ways. Talking is one of the normal developmental milestones that parents anticipate beginning at about age two; the absence of this milestone causes the reemergence of grief about the handicap. Also, because communication is the cornerstone of human relationships, the absence of this particular milestone has major implications for the parent/child relationship. Parents feel it intensely when their child is unable to tell them "I feel sick" or "I had a great time in school" or "I love you." Moreover, parents who are thinking of the future may recognize that lack of speech will affect the child's interpersonal relationships for the rest of his or her life.

To accept not talking, then, is to accept a whole new dimension of the handicap. This in itself brings its own grief reaction. The ability of parents to accept the use of a communication system and work with professionals will depend to a great extent on the parents' emotional state. An assessment of the parents' stage of grieving provides guidance to the professionals about the most effective approach to involving the parents. Professionals must remember that these feelings and responses are not discrete, and do not get resolved and disappear. They should be prepared for reemergence of a variety of feelings, particularly at the time of the introduction of the need for an augmentative communication system. Making parents active members of the evaluation and treatment team can facilitate realistic acceptance of the child's condition and serves the parents' immediate need of improved communication with their child. Providing parents with input and decision-making power in the design of the system reduces the distance between parent and "professional" and gives parents an element of control in the child's treatment; symbolically this empowers parents who may feel helpless to influence their child's future. Involving parents directly thus contributes to the child's use of an augmentative communication system by ensuring that they support use of the system, both because it is of practical use to them and because they are emotionally invested in the process.

Along with the social/emotional assessment of the family, professionals need to know what type of communication process is already used within the family, what information can be successfully communicated and what are the unmet communication needs. Communication interaction patterns between parents and nonspeaking children are likely to differ from the norm. Light, Collier and Parnes[11] analyzed the interaction patterns of eight congenitally nonspeaking physically disabled children between four and six years of age and their primary caregivers, from observations made during 20 minute free play situations. Data were analyzed to reflect the frequencies of the specific communicative behaviors of the participants and the patterns of interactional sequences within the conversations. Results indicated that the interaction patterns were transactional in nature, with caregivers and children clearly influencing each other in the course of the exchanges. Shared responsibility for communication was absent, however, as the communicaton process was clearly dominated by the caregivers. These authors suggested that early intervention is necessary to facilitate development of communication and social interaction skills if the goal is communicative competence and independence. To be effective, early intervention strategies must consider the interaction patterns of both the caregiver and the child. They suggested that caregivers be encouraged to attend to the informational aspects of communication as well as the structural aspects. Further encouragement is necessary to enhance development of realistic expectations for their nonverbal child and gradually yield responsibility for communication interaction to the child. As intervention is recommended, parents will need attention and guidance in figuring out how to combine their already established system of communication with the new one, e.g., when can they appropriately use the new system? How can it be made accessible when the child is with the family? One publication directed specifically to parental education and involvement techniques is the *Parent Training Manual*, edited by J. Kahane,[12] as a result of Project TEACH: Technical Education Aids for Children with Handicaps, Memphis, Tennessee. The manual describes the parent education and involvement techniques used in this project.

Strategies with Families

As professionals are assessing families, they are also guiding families through the augmentative communication evaluation process. Parents must be given basic information prior to learning about all options. Introduction and use of the words "augmentative communication" is in itself novel for families. In 1984-86 Altheide and Hough[13] conducted a nationwide survey of parents of non-verbal children and found that over 65% of the 100 parents surveyed did not initially know the meaning of the words "augmentative communication." Parents generally request basic information concerning the evaluation, selection, funding, training and use of an augmentative communication system or device. As members of the interdisciplinary assessment team, parents can benefit from guidance throughout the evaluation process and device trials. Providing ongoing commentary as parents observe can increase awareness of the strengths and weaknesses of their child's cognitive and motor performance and will assist parents in understanding the components of the evaluation and the recommendations which follow.

When an augmentative communication system or device is recommended, a common parental misconception is that the professionals (without telling the parents) are giving up on the child ever talking or that the augmentative communication system itself will prevent emergence of speech. These are such common responses that clarification should become a routine part of the initial discussion with parents regarding augmentative communication. Silverman[14] has reviewed extensive literature which supports the theory that teaching use of a nonspeech communication mode does not appear to reduce motivation for speech communication. Parents need to be told that use of a system will not inhibit speech; that, in fact, repeated frustration and inability to communicate is more likely to discourage a child. They need reassurance that the child will use speech when he or she can successfully communicate vocally. They should be gently reminded of the reality of the child's inability to communicate successfully vocally in at least some environments, and the need for an "augment" to speech should be discussed. Parents can understand that a system that "augments" speech prevents the child from becoming so frustrated that he or she "turns off" to communication. Parents also appreciate reassurance that, rather than inhibiting speech, an augmentative communication system often has very much the opposite effect—that the enthusiasm generated by successful communication generalizes to more investment in speech. The child will recognize that speech is the preferred (and easier) method of communication, and will use speech rather than an augment when speech is successful.

Discussion of what it may be like for the child to be unable to communicate with people who know the child less well is a useful way to assist parents in accepting the need for a system. Parents often say that they can communicate very well with their child, and in many ways they may be able to. Careful investigation into parent/child communication, however, can usually elicit areas in which the child is unable to communicate information to the parent, or to express important information to others. Exploring how well the child communicates with other people (teachers, extended family, babysitters) is informative to parents. Most parents have concerns about their child communicating important information to people other than themselves, such as telling the teacher that he or she is sick, or asking to use the bathroom. It is often useful to ask parents how the child would describe to them an event that happened at school that day. Beukelman[15] describes this as "information exchange across environmental boundaries." The child may be able to communicate within the family about family-related topics, and communicate within the school environment about school-related subjects and events, but without a point of reference may have no way to introduce new topics to a new environment. A thoughtful discussion of the child's communication needs can usually uncover some area of communication in which the parents would like improvement, and they are more likely to be invested in a system that facilitates communication on these topic areas.

Many alternative strategies are available for interacting with families about these concerns. In late 1985, the Center for Development and Learning at the University of North Carolina[16] surveyed University Affiliated Programs and 10 additional Augmentative Communication Evaluation Centers to determine the current status of information and services provided to families of augmentative communication users. Survey results indicated that the initial explanation of the concept of augmentative communication to the client's family was generally conducted through verbal discussion, sometimes supplemented with written information. Demonstration was an additional strategy, thus allowing characteristics of actual devices to be viewed. Providing demonstration and hands-on access to the equipment reportedly generated interest and questions. Although the majority of facilities surveyed utilized an interdisciplinary process for evaluation, the survey indicated that speech pathologists generally had primary responsibility for the explanation of augmentative communication to the family.

Once the concept of augmentative communication has been presented and explained to parents, the professionals can expect parents to lean heavily on them for guidance about next steps. Anticipatory guidance, a means of prevention, is an approach that has gained recognition from physicians and in public health literature. The concept of anticipatory guidance suggests that there are opportune times to support and prepare parents. A multitude of questions and concerns will arise during the introduction of something new such as augmentative communication.[17] In this instance, anticipatory guidance could assist in preventing excess anxiety and emotional stress. This guidance involves professionals spending considerable direct contact time with parents and developing a supportive working relationship with the family. Although viewed as a systematic approach, anticipatory guidance allows for expression of characteristics and needs of the child. The primary goal is to foster a good relationship between the parent and child.

Parents are likely to seek and need guidance at certain predictable times. One such instance is parental observation of a device trial. During that session the clinical team members could: (1) explain the components of the device; (2) explain the process needed to activate the device; (3) discuss the user's performance; (4) allow parents hands-on experiences with the device while providing guidance and explanation; (5) incorporate time for parents to independently try operation of the device without professionals present; (6) allow time for questions; (7) discuss initial vocabulary: versatility and expandability; and (8) provide information about price, dealer, rental/purchase options, maintenance and repair, precautions, and warranty.

FUNDING CONSIDERATIONS

Funding of augmentative communication systems appears to be a concern which parents and professionals must address together. Altheide and Hough[13] found that of 100 parents surveyed over 75% did not know of agencies to contact for information on how to pay for their child's communication system or necessary training. The Center for Development and Learning's Servicces to Families Survey indicated that a wide variety of funding sources had been successful in purchasing communication systems. Service organizations ranked first, followed by private organizations and Vocational Rehabilitation. Other sources included third party payers such as Medicaid, Crippled Children's, educational funding, community fund raising, private foundations and community agencies, state money, private payment and trust funds. The majority of facilities encountered problems with funding and described the process as time consuming for professionals. Communication devices were found not to be covered as medically necessary and a constant need to appeal this decision was reported.

In order to document medical necessity the physician must write or sign the justification for purchase. In "High Technology for Handicapped Children: A Pediatrician's Viewpoint" Desch[18] discussed funding issues. He reviewed the role of the physician in obtaining funding for devices and discussed the three false impressions of funding sources concerning microcomputers and other electronic assistive devices which were previously identified by Vanderheiden[19]: (1) the view of technology as a cure, (2) the view of a microcomputer or electronic assistive device as a toy, and (3) lack of good application and delivery systems for technical aids. Desch pointed out that government health programs and third-party programs prefer to provide reimbursement for durable medical equipment that immediately helps the client. Assistive electronic devices do not so readily supply immediate results, although tremendous benefits do occur with time.

A variety of professionals have identified the necessity of providing well documented need statements supported by attending clinicians and accompanied by evaluation and trial use data. Regulations and financial limitations within funding sources mean that the agency must clearly identify that a need exists and that thorough evaluation has occurred. Need alone is not always sufficient. Desch noted research conducted by the Office of Technology Assessment (US Congressional Agency) which indicated that some physically disabled persons were denied funding for technologies that were clearly appropriate. The agency also found that in situations where funding was obtained, additional financial support for supportive services such as instruction in proper use, fitting, training, and maintenance was often excluded.

In *The Many Faces of Funding* Hofmann,[20] market research analyst for Phonic Ear, Inc., provides a procedures section which outlines steps for pursuing funding, as well as a checklist and strategies to consider in assembling supportive documents and building credibility. In monthly updates Hofmann reviews current methods and suggests new strategies to obtain funding.

Beukelman, Yorkston and Smith[21] conducted an 18 month survey of third party payer response to requests for purchase of communication augmentation equipment for communicatively impaired individuals in the State of Washington. A total of 53 requests were returned from 12 agencies. Seventy percent of the requests were approved and thirty percent rejected or deferred. The mean cost of approved systems was $878 and for those rejected was $1,324.

Given the current difficulties in obtaining funding, professionals need to explore alternatives for obtaining augmentative communication equipment for their clients. One example of such alternatives is the Assistive Device Loan Program, developed by the Pennsylvania Department of Education, Bureau of Special Education, to provide appropriate high technology, assistive device systems to handicapped students in intermediate units, school districts and approved schools. The systems are placed on long-term loan for individual student use in the classroom and at home. Due to the individual nature of each student's assistive device system, these loans are designated to individual students rather than to classrooms or itinerant teachers. The loaned system remains with the student for the duration of his or her affiliation with special education programs and services in Pennsylvania. Upon determination that a loaned system is not meeting the current needs of the designated student, the Local Education Agency representative may request that the student be re-evaluated to receive modifications or a different system. Any equipment which is not being utilized will be recalled by the Assistive Device Center for placement with another student. This method allows extended time for personal purchase of a device.

SUMMARY

Successful implementation of an augmentative communication system requires family involvement. This process involves assessment of strengths and stresses within the family and communication patterns within the family. Assistance in obtaining funding for purchase, programming and maintenance of devices must also be provided.

REFERENCES

1. Ad Hoc Committee on Communication Processes and Nonspeaking Persons: Nonspeech communication: A position statement. *Rehab World* 7(2):40-43, 1983.

2. Paul J (ed): *Understanding and Working with Parents of Children with Special Needs*. New York, Holt, Rinehart & Winston, 1981.

3. Montgomery J: *Non-Oral Communication: A Training Guide for the Child Without Speech*. Fountain Valley, CA, Fountain Valley School District, 1980.

4. Shane H, Bashir A: Election criteria for the adoption of an augmentative communication system: Preliminary considerations. *J Speech Hear Disord* 45:408-414, 1980.

5. Klein S: New voices: Communication through technology. *Except Parent* 13(3):18-26, 1983.

6. American Speech-Language-Hearing Association & United States Department of Education: *Implementation Strategies for Improving Use of Communication Aids in Schools Serving Handicapped Children*. 1985-86.

7. Goolsby E: Factors that determine family response to a child with developmental handicaps, unpublished manuscript, Division for Disorders of Development and Learning, University of North Carolina, Chapel Hill, NC, 1978.

8. Blacher J: Sequential stages of parental adjustment to the birth of a child with handicaps: Fact or artifact? *Ment Retard* 22(2):55-68, 1984.

9. Olshansky S: Chronic sorrow: A response to having a mentally defective child. *Social Casework* 43:190-193, 1962.

10. Wikler L: Chronic stresses of families of mentally retarded children, in Wikler L, Keenam M (eds): *Dev Disabil* Washington, NASW and AAMD, 1983.

11. Light J, Collier B, Parnes P: Communicative interaction between young nonspeaking physically disabled children and their primary caregivers: Part 1 – Discourse patterns, *Augment Altern Commun* 1(2):74-83, 1985.

12. Kahane J (ed): *Project TEACH: Technical Educational Aids for Children with Handicaps – A Parent Training Manual*, Memphis City Schools, Division of Special Education, Memphis, TN, 1981.

13. Altheide MR, Hough S: Augmentative communication: Parent needs assessment, unpublished survey, Division for Disorders of Development and Learning, University of North Carolina at Chapel Hill, 1984-86.

14. Silverman F: *Communication for the Speechless*. Englewood Cliffs, NJ, Prentice-Hall, 1980.

15. Beukelman D: Keynote address-Spring Meeting of the North Carolina Augmentative Communication Association, Greensboro, NC, March 1986.

16. Livermore J, Altheide MR, Goolsby E: Augmentative Communication Services to Families, unpublished survey, Clinical Center for the Study of Development and Learning, University of North Carolina, Chapel Hill, NC, 1985-86.

17. Altheide MR, Hough S: *Proposal for Development of Parent Information Packet on Augmen-*

tative Communication, unpublished manuscript. Maternal and Child Health Care Postgraduate Fellowship Project-Grant 149, Division of Physical Therapy, Department of Medical Allied Health Professions, School of Medicine, University of North Carolina, Chapel Hill, NC, Spring 1984.

18. Desch L: High technology for handicapped children: A pediatrician's viewpoint. *Pediatrics* 77(1):71-87, 1986.

19. Vanderheiden G: The practical use of microcomputers in rehabilitation. *Rehabil Lit* 44:66-70, 1983.

20. Hofmann A: *The Many Faces of Funding*, ed 3. Phonic Ear Inc., 1986.

21. Beukelman D, Yorkston K, Smith K: Third-party payer response to requests for purchase of communication augmentation systems: A study of Washington State. *Augment Altern Commun* 1(1):5-9, 1985.

Interaction Strategies

Carolyn Eddins

SUMMARY. Successful interaction with a nonverbal, physically handicapped child depends greatly on the conversational partner's knowledge of the child's communication system. This paper describes basic components of communicative interaction, and differences between spoken and nonverbal, augmented communication. Ways in which these differences influence interactions and strategies to facilitate communication with augmented communicators are discussed. Finally, a series of personal commentaries is presented.

INTRODUCTION

In the past decade, speech-language pathologists have recognized the development of communicative interaction skills as a primary goal of intervention with nonvocal, physically handicapped children using augmentative communication systems.[1-7] Simply providing these children with an augmentative system, however, does not ensure that they will become successful participants in communicative interactions.[4,7] Differences in the communication/interaction systems, processes and expertise of these children influence their choice of interaction partners; topics of communication; length, complexity and functions of messages and conversational turns; intelligibility, appropriateness, accuracy and completeness of messages; and responsibility and control assumed by the child during an interaction. Yoder and Kraat[6] identified five major variables which make the augmented communication of physically handicapped children different from the spoken communication of non-physically handicapped children. These are developmental constraints, expressive modes, symbol systems, rate of communication and interactive processes. Interaction partners who understand these differences and the affect they have on a child's ability to communicate will be better prepared to engage in successful interactions with the non-speaking child.

In this article a brief review of the major components of communicative interaction is presented, followed by a discussion of the differences imposed by augmented communication. Suggestions for enhancing the

Carolyn Eddins, MS, CCC-SP, Speech Pathology Department, Jackson Memorial Hospital, 1611 NW 12th Avenue, Miami, FL 33136.

quantity and quality of the child's interactions are provided. The paper concludes with a series of personal comments from communication system users and partners.

COMPONENTS OF COMMUNICATIVE INTERACTION

Successful communicative interaction depends on accurate transmission of messages between partners who share knowledge of the linguistic and nonlinguistic components of the messages. The ability to initiate or establish a topic by providing or requesting new information is also fundamental to successful interaction.[8] Following topic initiation, a partner's response offers feedback as to what information was actually transmitted and the effect it had on the receiver. If a message is not interpreted as the sender intended, a communication breakdown occurs which must be repaired before resuming the original topic. A response may set in motion a series of turns, thus maintaining the topic or initiating a new one,[9] or it may serve to terminate the topic and the interaction.

For most people, speech is the primary mode of communication; it provides a rapid means of verbal expression using a shared symbol system for speakers of a given language. The verbal, or linguistic, message, however, is only one component of the communicative interaction. Nonverbal behaviors also convey referential information (as in pointing and gestures) as well as attitudes, emotional states, and personal characteristics, and serve to regulate the flow of the interaction.[5,10,11] These nonverbal behaviors, discussed by Higginbotham and Yoder,[5] include:

1. *paralinguistics:* the vocal characteristics of pitch, intensity, articulation, stress and intonation patterns, and timing, which provide information about the speaker's background, personality, and emotional state;
2. *kinesics:* the body postures and movements which communicate affective state and need for attention, and opinions, and regulate turn-taking;
3. *proxemics:* the physical distance between interactants, used in initiating and terminating topics or conversations, in regulating turn taking, and as indicators of the degree of familiarity of the conversational partners; and
4. *chronemics:* the coordination of verbal and nonverbal modalities.

Skilled use of culturally meaningful verbal and nonverbal behaviors develops as one matures cognitively, linguistically and motorically.[2,12,13] These behaviors are reinforced by the effects they have on the user's environment. Among the purposes for which children communicate are to give information; request information; describe events; persuade listeners to do, believe or feel something; express intentions, feelings or beliefs; regulate interactions; entertain and learn new behaviors.[14,15]

DIFFERENCES AFFECTING THE COMMUNICATION OF NONVOCAL CHILDREN

Developmental Constraints

The physically handicapped child's limited mobility and motor control affect his or her capacity to "explore, manipulate, and experience objects, persons and events."[2(p234)] Cognitive, linguistic, social and communicative interaction skill development can be negatively influenced by the child's lack of consistent, volitional interaction with the environment. [2,3,6,13] Thus, the child approaches communicative interactions with limited experiences about which to communicate, little knowledge of interactive behaviors, decreased motivation to communicate and learned passivity and dependency based on prior experience.[2,6]

Harris and Vanderheiden encouraged those developing communication interaction intervention programs to "provide mechanisms and strategies to enable or enhance interaction."[2(p236)] Indeed, this can be viewed as a multi- or interdisciplinary goal. For example, appropriate positioning, development of fine and gross motor control, and adaptation of objects and situations increase the child's ability to experience and control the environment. Many types of intervention must be offered if the child is to realize his or her potential to interact with the environment.

Different Expressive Modes

The augmented communicator employs a multi-modal process for message production.[16] Expressive modes may include vocalization, limited intelligible verbalization, augmentative aids (i.e., communication boards and devices with visual and/or auditory output), signing, gestures, pointing, eye gaze, and nonverbal paralinguistic, kinesic and proxemic, behaviors.[5,16] Not all modalities are available to all children due to cognitive, motor and sensory impairment.[1,5,6] The successful production of any message requires the child to select his or her most efficient available mode(s) considering the familiarity and receptive sensory and linguistic ability of the intended receiver(s); the physical environment (i.e., level of ambient noise, available light); the accuracy and completeness with which the message can be formulated and produced via the chosen mode(s); and the function of the message within the context of the interaction.

Harris[4] and Light and colleagues[16] found that children tend to choose the fastest, most easily accessible, most familiar, and least physically demanding mode. Such choices may be inappropriate, placing additional responsibility for message interpretation on partners and leading to communication breakdowns, increased frustration and decreased motivation to communicate. For example, this occurs when an idiosyncratic gesture is used with an unfamiliar partner[6] or when asynchronous vocalization and eye gaze confuse the message receiver.[3,5]

Light and colleagues[16] identified diverse individual preferences in modes, or combinations of modes, used by the eight children they observed interacting with primary caregivers. The group trends, however, indicated a correlation between expressive mode and communicative function. They observed that children initiated topics most frequently by auditory or combined auditory and visual modes. These authors subsequently reported that while the children obtained their partner's attention in 85% of initiation attempts, they usually failed to adequately establish the topic and had to rely on partner elaboration of their messages.[7] Additionally, they reported that: (a) responses to previous messages with a shared topic or focus were accomplished in a vocalization, by board use, or by gesture; (b) information was provided by use of communication boards; (c) confirmation and denial (yes/no responses) were conveyed through vocalization or gestures; (d) clarification generally occurred through use of communication boards; and (e) requests for objects and actions were most likely to be produced by gesture and vocalization, eye gaze and vocalization. The children used communication boards for this purpose when cued to use them or when the objects being discussed were not visible.[16] These authors concluded that, in general, the children they observed employed context-appropriate modes of expression.

Harris[4] suggested that interaction partners may need to encourage children to use their most effective modes, but that communication through any modality should be accepted if the message is adequately conveyed. Ideally, the child would have access to all modes at all times, but this is not always possible.[8] In an active treatment setting, all of the expressive modes used by a child may not be readily available to him or her. When the child is removed from the wheelchair, the communication board or device is generally left behind. Pointing, gestures or eye gaze may be inconsistent or impossible when the child is in certain therapeutic positions. Yet children need to interact with their therapists to increase familiarity, rapport and motivation; to communicate basic needs and novel experiences; and to further develop overall interaction skills.

Therapists can encourage use of any one mode, particularly a communication board or device, by providing time at the beginning, during, and after treatment sessions when the mode is available to the child. For example, special signals devised by therapist and child could allow the child access to a board or device during therapy to provide information or repair communication breakdowns.

Morris[3] and Higginbotham and Yoder[5] advocate improving the quality of whatever modalities are available to the child at any given time. Training a child with inconsistent vocalization to use eye gaze to different areas in the room, to look up versus down, or to use one eye blink versus two, might provide him or her with a way to indicate yes or no responses during therapy activities. Pointing or eye gaze can be employed to make choices after the therapist has raised one hand while verbalizing choice A and the other hand while verbalizing choice B. Accurate feedback from the therapist as to the message conveyed by a child's facial expression can help the child improve use of that modality.

Different Symbol Systems

Closely related to the expressive modes employed by a child are the symbol systems he or she uses. Written words, the alphabet (for letter-by-letter spelling), pictures, real objects, finger spelling and sign language, Morse code, and special systems, such as Rebus and Blissymbolics, have been coupled with a variety of expressive modes. These nonoral symbol systems pose two major barriers to interaction – vocabulary is restricted and the number of potential partners is limited.[4,6,17]

Vocabulary restrictions are imposed for a variety of reasons. Certainly cognitive and linguistic impairments limit the number of vocabulary items employed by some children. Yet even these children may experience additional expressive restrictions when using augmentative systems. On many communication boards or devices, space limitations exist due to mobility and portability factors [6] and the child's range of motion for accessing symbols. Children who spell messages letter-by-letter or through finger spelling are limited by their spelling skills. Children who communicate through sign language are limited to using the signs that they can physically produce and those they have learned. These may be relatively few in number unless they live in a community where others employ sign language as a primary symbol system.

Limitation of vocabulary items affects the quality of the message transmitted during an interaction.[4] Yoder and Kraat [6] discussed the inability of the child's expressive vocabulary to change rapidly enough to reflect cognitive and receptive language development. Thus, the child may be unable to convey information about recent experiences and new topics, to use the latest slang expressions, or to engage in linguistic development through experimentation and play with symbols.[4,6] Children often lack the symbols needed to express complete intent; they must then condense a number of meanings into a one or two symbol message that merely approximates, but does not fully convey the desired message. Alternatively, the child might choose to refrain from communicating to avoid the frustration of an inaccurate or incomplete message.

Interaction partners have been observed to make assumptions about a child's cognitive and linguistic development based on expressive skills that are limited by the available vocabulary or symbol system.[6] This prompts partners to immaturize their speech, as when talking to a young child,[17] or to fail to expand messages as needed.[4] Accurate information about a child's receptive and expressive level can be obtained through observation of the child's interactions with objects and persons in the environment and from caregivers and professionals familiar with him or her.

Successful communicative interaction frequently depends on the partner's ability to elaborate on the child's messages. For example, the 20-questions method,[17] a series of yes or no questions moving from general to specific, might help a partner determine that the symbols "food" and "go" mean "We're going out to eat tonight." Following elaborations, the child should provide feedback on the accuracy of the partner's interpretation; if the child fails to offer this, the partner needs to check with the child to assure accurate interpretation of the message. Partners may need to offer the child choices of words to ascertain true intent, particularly when the appropriate symbols are not available.

A restricted expressive vocabulary and the type of symbol system(s) employed by a child limit potential interaction partners.[6] Some partners are not familiar enough with certain topics as they relate to the child to adequately expand the messages produced with a limited vocabulary.[6] Nonreaders experience limited interaction with children who use an alphabet or word board. Untrained partners may be unable to interact successfully with children who use finger spelling or sign language. Special symbol systems designed for augmentative communication (i.e., Rebus and Blissymbolics) are not readily comprehensible to all partners.[6]

To address this problem, Yoder and Kraat[6] suggested developing multiple symbol systems and vocabularies for use in different environments. For example, a fifth grade student might use an alphabet/word board at school while a picture/alphabet/word board, could be used at home to facilitate interaction with younger siblings.

An understanding of the symbol system(s) used by a child and the limitations they impose enables those interacting with the child to help him or her develop better interactive skills within the system constraints; to determine appropriate vocabulary additions and deletions; and to recognize the need for new or additional systems as the child develops cognitively, linguistically, socially and motorically.

Different Rate of Communication

The use of augmentative communication systems imposes a reduced rate of communication when compared to the use of speech. The type of system employed and the augmented communicator's physical abilities influence the rate at which a message is generated and received.[6,18] The process of message production is less automatic and more complex for the augmentative system user than for one using speech. For example, a child communicating the linguistic aspects of a message via an alphabet/word board must decide what he or she wants to communicate; determine which aspects of the message can be transmitted by nonlinguistic or nonverbal behaviors; identify which words are readily available on the board and which must be spelled out; obtain the partner's visual attention; visually locate and motorically indicate each word or letter needed; indicate to the partner when words or messages are complete; and exchange feedback with the partner to assure accurate reception of each component of the message. Much effort is required to produce a message, and under stressful conditions the child's motor control can be compromised, thereby increasing the time and energy needed for message production.[4]

Decreased rate of communication has many ramifications for communicative interactions. Harris[4] reported a tendency to sacrifice message accuracy for increased speed of production, thus increasing the likelihood of communication breakdowns. Children have been observed to produce fewer messages per conversational turn than do their partners, or to use telegraphic output (substantive words/symbols, usually nouns and verbs) which the partner must expand into complete messages. They may opt for producing no message rather than one that might be irrelevant to the interaction or event by the time it is transmitted to the partner.[4,6] The decreased rate also makes difficult the synchronization of linguistic elements with the non-linguistic behaviors of the child and partner.[5]

Many children and their partners experience frustration due to the decreased rate of communication. Compounding this frustration are attempts to speed up the process which result in communication breakdowns requiring additional time and energy to repair. Partners often attempt prediction of a message based on initial letter or word sequences. Beukelman and Yorkston[19] found that familiarity with partners seemed to influence success of message prediction. They suggested that "strangers or less familiar partners usually find communication easier if they confirm the portion of the message they understand rather than attempt to add new information".[18(p 44)] Partners are advised to ask the child if he or she desires message prediction, and to bear in mind that over-anticipation or expansion of a child's message promotes dependency versus responsibility for the communicative interaction. All of these authors encouraged devising a signal by which the child can provide feedback as to the accuracy of the partner's prediction.

Partners have also been noted to inundate a child with a series of yes or no questions during periods of message formulation. Instead of increasing the overall rate of communication, this can distract and confuse the child and is just as rude and inappropriate as it would be if the questions were directed to someone while speaking. Interaction partners must learn to be patient and to wait for the child to produce messages. Harris[4] reported that when partners allow adequate time for message generation and transmission, children appear to produce complex messages as opposed to one word or yes/no responses. This serves to decrease the possibility of communication breakdown and to increase the child's active participation in the interaction.

Different Interaction Processes

Nonvocal physically handicapped children approach communication interactions with constraints that alter the usual patterns of conversation and necessitate the use of unconventional styles and strategies to achieve successful interaction.[4,6] The child often has difficulty initiating conversational interactions, and several turns may be devoted simply to establishing the topic. The child might also need assistance in maintaining conversation, changing topics, and terminating an interaction. Light and colleagues[7] reported that the children they observed required increased time to initiate topics and, indeed, were infrequent initiators. These children took an average of one half as many turns as did their partners, and one half as many as were available to them. They were most likely to respond when the partner's previous message demanded a response and when a minimal response would suffice. Thus, the reciprocity, timing and content of initiation and response turns were unlike that in spoken interactions.

Farrier and associates cited numerous studies of conversational control in interactions between non-vocal children and vocal partners. They defined conversational control as "the manner and extent to which an individual directs or restrains communicative interaction."[20(p65)] In general, studies of conversational control find children to be in minimal control of the content and flow of interactions. Variables contributing to their lack of control include: the type of augmentative communication system used and the need for partner involvement in message production and interpretation;[18,21,22] conversational experience;[4] cognitive and linguistic abilities;[6] rate and timing of message production[20] and familiarity of partners.[5] Conversational control can be increased by building into the child's communication system special signals or phrases to indicate the completion of a conversational turn, the need for more time (i.e., raised hand, "Please wait"), and so forth. This will provide the child with the ability to compensate for some inconsistent or absent nonverbal behaviors.[5]

Communication frequently breaks down during interactions involving augmented communicators. Breakdowns and subsequent repairs alter the natural flow of conversation. Partners can increase a child's conversational responsibility by learning to facilitate repair rather than feigning comprehension when communication breaks down. Some repair strategies are partner-dependent, such as the 20-question method and use of multiple choice questions. Others are child-dependent: changing expressive modes and paraphrasing or repeating the message. Partners may need to cue the child to use his or her most efficient strategy. Repairs take time; they can become so frustrating that it is appropriate to move on to another topic, but only with the child's permission. The partner's willingness to pursue repair conveys to the child the importance of his or her messages, thereby reinforcing communication.

INTERACTION SUGGGESTIONS FOR PARTNERS

There are many ways in which partners can facilitate increased conversational participation by a child. Some of these have already been mentioned. Other suggestions for partners include:

- —communicate with the child, not just with others accompanying him or her;
- —ask questions which require elaborate responses rather than yes/no or one word messages;[22]
- —allow the child to direct the partner in completion of tasks;[2]
- —encourage the child to interact with peers;[4]
- —communicate with the child for pleasure, so that he or she can express a variety of thoughts, emotions and communication functions;[4]
- —encourage initiation of topics and interactions by staying close to the child[22] and maintaining visual contact with him or her;[23]
- —teach a child to obtain others' attention and offer sufficient information to establish a topic;[7]
- —provide ample time, opportunity and need to initiate conversation; and
- —follow up on non-verbal leads.

PERSONAL PERSPECTIVES

The strategies just described require time and energy, especially in the first stages of a developing relationship. Clearly there is no single formula for going about the process, and both partners must invest time and energy as well as take emotional risks. To illustrate these points, comments have been elicited from four individuals who have extensive personal experience with augmentative communication. Each was asked to address a specific issue, and their responses are offered here for the benefit of the readers.

Born in Smithfield, North Carolina, Rick Creech was one of the first users of a portable vocal output communication aid. Mr. Creech has contributed to several augmentative communication publications and is presently the editor of the Min-Speak Corp. newsletter. He graduated Magna Cum Laude from East Carolina University with a BA in English. He is a business writer and lives in Richmond, VA. He was asked to discuss the emotional components of interacting with users of communication systems.

Mr. Creech: The usual reaction to communicating with a speech impaired person is nervous anxiety. Some people will avoid contact with an augmented speaker because they cannot overcome their anxiety, or should I say, fear. Most of my friends have confessed to being anxious, afraid, scared stiff when they first met me.

Anxious fear is normal when we are expected to perform well in a difficult situation. The augmented speaker needs to keep in mind that this "fear" is not a reaction to him or her as a person, but results from the other's insecurity about being able to interact with a speech impaired individual. The augmented speaker has a compound problem of calming the fears of others while dealing with his or her own fears about interacting and being able to communicate with people.

In order not to take this reaction of people personally, the augmented speaker needs to be able to separate himself or herself from his or her disability and accept a negative reaction to the disability as only that and not as reaction to the person. When the speech impaired person does this, he or she will be able to help the other person become comfortable in the interacting.

The first step the augmented speaker must take in helping a person is to initiate a conversation. The speech impaired person must put others in a situation that compels them to speak. I usually accomplish this by driving my wheelchair in front of a person and sitting there until the person says, "May I help you?" This is a little impolite, but sometimes it does not pay to be too polite.

The second step is to show patience. Communicating with an augmented speaker is more frustrating for the other person than it is for the augmented speaker because the person using a communication aid has had experience in augmented speech, whereas it may be the other person's first experience with augmented communication. Patience often may run low, but letting patience run out rarely pays.

The third step is to smile. This may sound like trite advice, but it works. In order for an augmented speaker to get people to interact with him or her, the speaker must attract people, and smiles attract people. The speech impaired individual may be very intelligent, a great conversationalist, and an interesting person, but unless he or she is advertising a good personality with a smile, people will not make the extra effort to communicate.

Some people cannot overcome their fear of the disability and are never able to interact with the person within. The speech impaired person cannot interact with these people because they run from the augmented speaker. They avoid eye contact, mumble, shift weight from one foot to another, and show every sign of wanting to flee. In this case the person with the handicap is not the one who uses an augmented speaking device. The handicapped person is the one who cannot communicate.

Sara Carter is a Speech-Language Pathologist at the Clinical Center for the Study of Development and Learning at the University of North Carolina at Chapel Hill. She has both devised and utilized communication systems for clients of all ages, and has an unusual ability to establish rapport with them. She was asked to comment on two areas of the communication process.

Ms. Eddins: What do you think about when you begin an interaction with a non-verbal child?

Ms. Carter: I immediately assume an attitude of personal intimacy, an attitude that I can know that person well. I also simply make a decision that time is of no consequence. That is, "efficiency" is not important to our communicative interaction. I also assume that the non-verbal person will benefit from openness and honesty with me. I immediately make them a confidante, if I can, by saying something personal about myself. I try to let them know as soon as possible that I am available to them as a communicating person. I look at them. And let them look at me—a large, extended "hello."

Ms. Eddins: Do you worry about getting stuck, about not knowing what they are trying to say?

Ms. Carter: You mean, do I worry about failing? No, I don't. I assume that the two of us will have failures in our attempts to exchange information. I'm not worried about that. What I worry about is that nothing will happen between us, nothing of interest to either of us. So I usually begin by asking a question I want an answer to. Something like, "How did you get that gash on your head?" or "Where do you keep this chair when you're not sitting in it?" or "Do you know why you're here?"

I think it's critical to ask questions you don't have the answers to. That's what makes communication so much fun: getting and giving information you haven't had before. When each person in the communication act is merely exchanging "known information," then there's not much pleasure in the process.

I also have an idea about the usefulness of failures with nonverbal persons. I think that failing can be a shared experience; both of you know that something was intended that didn't get conveyed. And you hold in trust that you will be able to find out eventually or that something just as important will eventually be exchanged because both parties are willing to put in a good effort. It's possible, even with failure, to build up trust between the two people and trust is one of the finest exchanges that can occur between human beings.

Bruce Baker, of Pittsburgh, Pennsylvania is a neurolinguist, consultant to Prentke Romich Company, and creator of Min-Speak, a computer-based language retrieval system for augmentative communication devices. He was asked to comment on the unique characteristics of augmented communication.

Mr. Baker: When an ablebodied individual communicates with a person who uses a communication aid, the conversation develops in many ways that are typical for all conversations and in certain important ways that are different from typical conversations. These "different ways" make certain demands on both conversational partners and are the subject of these brief comments.

One of the most important "different ways" is that a means of confirmation is often needed between conversational partners that is not needed in a typical conversation. Let us say Mr. Jones who has cerebral palsy and uses a headstick and a manual board for communication purposes is having a conversation with a recent acquaintance named Ms. Smith. When Mr. Jones indicates a particular letter on his board with his headstick, his eyes are naturally directed down to the board. At that moment he is unable to tell whether Ms. Smith has noticed which letter he has selected. Unless Ms. Smith calls out the letter Mr. Jones has indicated, the conversation will soon founder. Neither party will know exactly what's going on.

This is only one example of the need for confirmation when alternative communication systems are being used. One special skill that Mr. Jones has to develop is to teach all new conversational partners his own confirmation system and having taught them, to keep them consistent until they have internalized this special feature of communicating with him.

Other types of alternative communication systems have their own special confirmation processes. Silent systems, whether manual or electronic, need more confirmation than do voice output systems. As voice quality improves with technological advances, the confirmation needs with voice systems will diminish. But improvement in voice quality is no panacea. It is the slowness and the time differences that make confirmation in voice systems necessary. So long as a particular voice system allows its users to generate speech only at very slow rates, some kind of confirmation system will remain necessary with a voice system no matter how human its quality. Readers can test this for themselves by conducting a conversation and hesitating 10 seconds between each word. Both conversational partners will soon need elaborate cross checks to monitor "where they are" in the conversation.

The length of time involved in a conversation using alternative communication systems is a primary factor in their differentness. The other primary factor applies only to silent systems, and that is that they are not conducted audibly. If an ablebodied individual wishes to become skilled in speaking with users of alternative communication systems whether silent or voiced, he or she is going to have to deal sooner or later with this time difference.

Scott Peck in his popular book entitled *The Road Less Traveled* mentions the idea that "caring is taking time." The truth of the statement is nowhere more evident than when an ablebodied person is speaking to someone who uses a communication aid. If I, as an ablebodied individual, am going to have a personal relationship whether business or social with a person using a communication system, I must be willing to manifest my caring by taking the time it takes to talk with someone who uses such an aid. It's as simple as that.

The role of the communication aid user is to minimize the time differential and to help his conversational partners, particularly inexperienced ones, deal with the anxiety that those time differences cause. It is the role of the communication aid developer to put enough linguistic power into the communication aid that the users have at their disposal the language they need to perform their role.

Lara Parker is a high school student in Dallas, Texas. She has athetoid cerebral palsy, and has used augmented communication systems since early childhood. She used her Autocom to offer this advice to therapists and teachers.

Ms. Parker: Working with a person who cannot speak may be very difficult for both the therapist or teacher and the individual who cannot talk. It is often mistakenly thought that a nonverbal person is not capable of making decisions directly affecting himself. This is untrue most of the time. Here are several pointers that will make working with a person who cannot speak easier and much more productive.

The first important pointer is for a therapist or teacher to understand completely why the student cannot speak. There are many possibilities. For instance, a student may have cerebral palsy which is damage to the brain that occurs before, during or soon after birth. The brain damage may cause a person to not be able to speak. In order for a therapist or teacher to understand why a student is nonverbal the following two steps are important. A meeting with the teacher from the year before is a step. During this meeting a teacher will learn how it feels to have a student who cannot speak in the class. Also, the previous year's teacher can tell how he included the nonverbal student in labs and group work. Another step in order to fully understand why the student cannot speak is to have a meeting with the student, his parents and if the student has an aide, the aide. They will explain why he is nonverbal, and how the student communicates. Also this meeting serves as an opportunity for the teacher to become comfortable around the student. These meetings should take place before school starts. For therapists there are two steps to follow in order to fully understand why the person is nonverbal. First, contact with the old therapist because he can tell what kinds of things to work on. A meeting with the person and his parents before therapy begins is another step. Understanding why the student is nonverbal is very important.

The next pointer for a therapist or teacher to be successful in working with a nonverbal person is to treat the person who cannot speak like a regular human being, not like a little poor crippled person who does not have any feelings. Treating a person who cannot speak like a normal person lets the nonverbal person know that the therapist or teacher recognizes him for what he can do, not what he cannot do. This is the key for a good working relationship between the nonverbal person and the therapist or teacher. Treating a person who cannot speak like a regular human being is very important to be more productive in working with a nonverbal person.

The third important pointer for the therapist or teacher in order to work with a nonverbal person successfully is methods to communicate with a person who cannot speak. The first method is signs either from sign language or signs which the nonverbal person and the therapist or teacher agree upon. For example, when the person who cannot speak points to his mouth, it might mean that he wants a drink. The second method is a communication board which can be manual or computerized. If the board is manual, the person needs the therapist or teacher to watch while he indicates. If the nonverbal person has a computerized board, the therapist or teacher will be free to do something else until the person who cannot speak lets him know when to look. With a communication board the person who cannot speak can express more complex thoughts. The third method of communication is yes/no. For example, if a therapist or teacher asks the nonverbal student a question like "Does red and blue make purple?", the therapist or teacher says "If yes, raise your hand", and "If no, shake your head." This method requires a criteria. The final method is multiple choice. For instance, if the therapist or teacher asks the person who cannot speak a question like "What is the name of this object?", the therapist or teacher says "a is a head, b is a hand or c is a chest." The nonverbal person indicates a, b or c by his communication board or yes/no. Including the nonverbal student in a class discussion may be difficult. These following suggestions might help. The first suggestion is to tell the person who cannot speak the question beforehand so that he can work on it without holding the rest of the class up. Giving the student who cannot speak multiple choice is another suggestion. The third suggestion is to ask the nonverbal student if a statement is true or false. Communication between the person who cannot speak and the therapist or teacher is very important.

The next pointer in order to make work with a nonverbal person more productive is for a therapist or teacher to be flexible. The nonverbal student may take longer to complete work than the rest of the class because he cannot communicate the answers as fast as the other students write. These following ways are designed to get the same concept from the student who cannot speak in a reasonable amount of time. The first way is if the assignment was to write the whole sentence and put in the correct verb tense, have the nonverbal student only write the correct verb. Or, if the student has an aide, have the aide write the sentence down, and the student who cannot speak will tell what verb to put in. If a test is taking the nonverbal student too long, pick out a portion that has to be done. If the student who cannot speak finishes early, have him do more. Grade what is done. If a therapist or teacher feels like the nonverbal student is getting lazy, increase the work load. Being flexible is very important for a good working relationship between the therapist or teacher and the nonverbal student.

Working with a nonverbal person may seem difficult at first. If a therapist or teacher will keep these four pointers in mind while working with a person who cannot speak, it will be a piece of cake!

NOTES

1. Harris-Vanderheiden D, Vanderheiden G: Basic considerations in the development of communicative and interactive skills of nonvocal severely handicapped children, in E Sontag, J Smith, N Certo (eds): *Educational Programming for the Severely/Profoundly Handicapped*. Reston, VA Council for Exceptional Children, 1977.

2. Harris D, Vanderheiden G: Enhancing the development of communicative interaction, in R Schiefelbusch (ed): *Nonspeech Language and Communication: Analysis and Intervention*. Baltimore, University Park Press, 1980.

3. Morris S: Communication/interaction development at mealtimes for the multiply handicapped child: Implications for the use of augmentative communication systems. *Language, Speech, and Hearing Services in Schools* 12: 216-232, 1981.

4. Harris D: Communicative interaction processes involving nonvocal physically handicapped children. *Topics in Language Disorders* 2: 21-37, 1982.

5. Higginbotham D, Yoder D: Communication within natural conversational interaction: Impli-

cations for severely communicatively impaired persons. *Topics in Language Disorders* 2: 1-19, 1982.

6. Yoder D, Kraat A: Intervention issues in nonspeech communication, in J Miller, D Yoder, R Schiefelbusch (eds): *Contemporary Issues in Communication Intervention*. ASHA Reports 12, 1983.

7. Light J, Collier B, Parnes P: Communicative interaction between young nonspeaking physically disabled children and their primary caregivers: Part I – Discourse patterns. *Augmentative and Alternative Communication* 1: 74-83, 1985.

8. Keenan E, Schiefflin B: Topic as a discourse notion: A study of topic in the conversations of children and adults, in C Li (ed): *Subject and Topic*. New York, Academic Press, 1976.

9. Bloom L, Rocissano L, Hood L: Adult-child discourse: Developmental interaction between information processing and linguistic knowledge. *Cognitive Psychology* 8: 521-552, 1976.

10. Argyle M: Non-verbal communication in human social interaction, in RA Hinde (ed): *Non-Verbal Communication*. Cambridge, England, Cambridge University Press, 1972.

11. Knapp M: *Nonverbal Communication in Human Interaction*. New York, Holt, Rinehart and Winston, 1978.

12. Piaget J: *The Origins of Intelligence in Children*. New York, WW Norton and Co, 1964.

13. Chapman R, Miller J: Analyzing language and communication in the child, in R Schiefelbusch (ed): *Nonspeech Language and Communication: Analysis and Intervention*. Baltimore, University Park Press, 1980.

14. Montgomery J: Measuring communication aid effectiveness. *Non-oral Communication Center Newsletter* 3: 1-3, 1980.

15. Musselwhite C, St. Louis K: *Communication Programming For the Severely Handicapped: Vocal and Non-vocal Strategies*. San Diego, College-Hill Press, 1980.

16. Light J, Collier B, Parnes P: Communicative interaction between young nonspeaking physically handicapped children and their primary caregivers: Part III – Modes of communication. *Augmentative and Alternative Communication* 1: 125-133, 1985.

17. Shane H, Cohen C: A discussion of communicative strategies and patterns by nonspeaking persons. *Language, Speech, and Hearing in Schools* 12: 205-210, 1981.

18. Beukelman D, Yorkston K: Communication interaction of adult communication augmentation system use. *Topics in Language Disorders* 2: 39-53, 1982.

19. Beukelman D, Yorkston K: Non-vocal communication – performance evaluation. *Arch Phys Med Rehabil*, 61: 272-275, 1980.

20. Farrier L, Yorkston K, Marriner N, Beakelman D: Conversational control in nonimpaired speakers using an augmentative communication system. *Augmentative and Alternative Communication* 2: 65-73, 1985.

21. Buzolich M: *Interaction analysis of augmented and normal adult communicators*, Doctoral dissertation. University of California, San Francisco, 1983.

22. Calculator S, Luchko C: Evaluating the effectiveness of a communication board training program. *Journal of Speech and Hearing Disorders* 48: 185-191, 1983.

23. Kraat A, Miller M: Hey you, I've got something to say: A study of the attention getting ability of a nonspeaking, physically disabled preschooler. Read before the Third International Conference on Augmentative and Alternative Communication, Boston, Mass, 1984.

APPENDIX I: RECORD FORMS FOR AUGMENTATIVE COMMUNICATION EVALUATION

Form A(1)

EYE GAZE SYSTEM

NAME: ____________ DATE: ____________ FAMILY ADVISOR: ____________

DOB: ____________ NCMH # ____________ COMMUNITY ADVOCATE: ____________

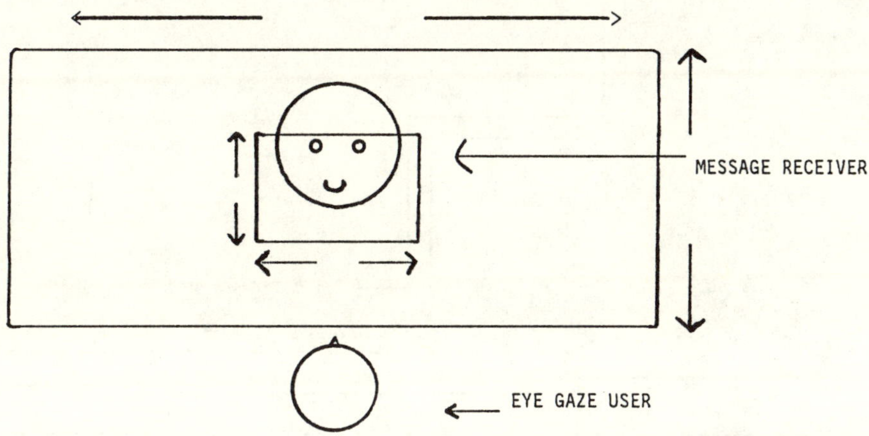

PLEXIGLASS SHEET

DIMENSIONS: ____________

SIZE OF CUTOUT: ____________

TYPE OF SYMBOLS TO BE DISPLAYED: ____________

SIZE OF SYMBOLS: ____________

NUMBER OF SYMBOLS TO BE DISPLAYED: ____________

PLACEMENT OF SYMBOLS: ____________

SIMPLE EYE GAZE SYSTEM USE:

1) EYE GAZE SYSTEM USER LOOKS CENTER

2) EYE GAZE SYSTEM USER LOOKS AT SELECTION DESIRED

3) EYE GAZE SYSTEM USER LOOKS BACK TO CENTER CUTOUT

Form A(2)

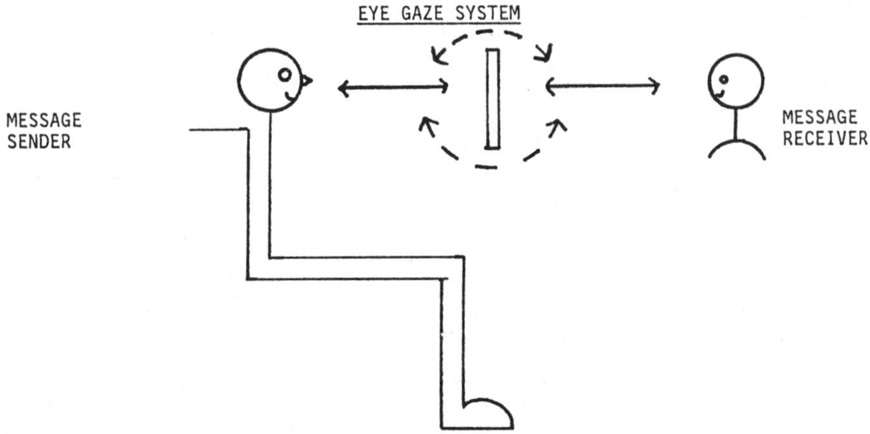

DISTANCE FROM USER'S FACE:________________________

DISTANCE FROM SENDER'S FACE:________________________

ANGLE:________________________

MOUNTING OPTIONS:________________________

____

____

____

ADDITIONAL COMMENTS:

RESOURCES:

Form B(1)

EYE GAZE SYSTEM WITH ENCODING

NAME:______________________________ DATE:______________

DOB:______________________ NCMH #______________

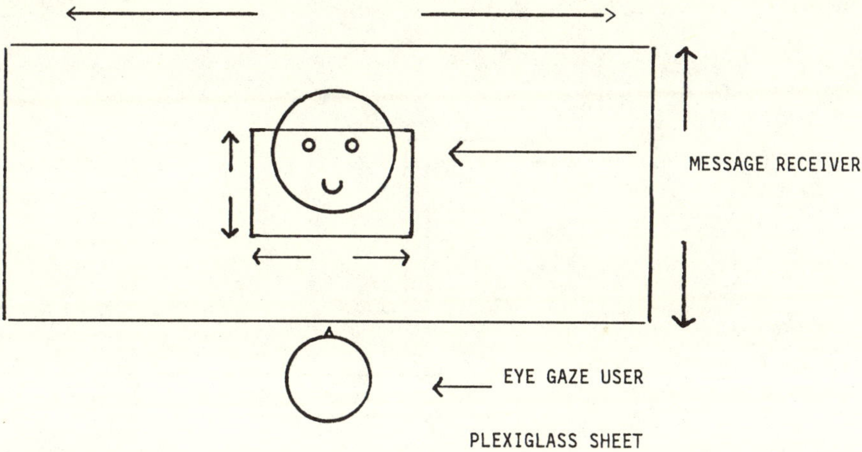

ENCODING SYSTEM:______________________
____
____
____
____

EXPANSION OF ENCODING SYSTEM:
____
____
____
____
____
____

DIMENSIONS:______________________

SYMBOLS TO BE DISPLAYED:__________
____

NUMBER OF SYMBOLS:______________

PLACEMENT OF SYMBOLS:___________

SIZE OF CUTOUT:_________________

USE OF EYE GAZE ENCODED SYSTEM:

1) USER LOOKS CENTER
2) USER LOOKS AT LOCATION
3) USER LOOKS CENTER
4) USER LOOKS TO INDICATE LOCATION SYMBOL WITHIN THE FIRST AREA SELECTED
5) USER LOOKS CENTER

Form B(2)

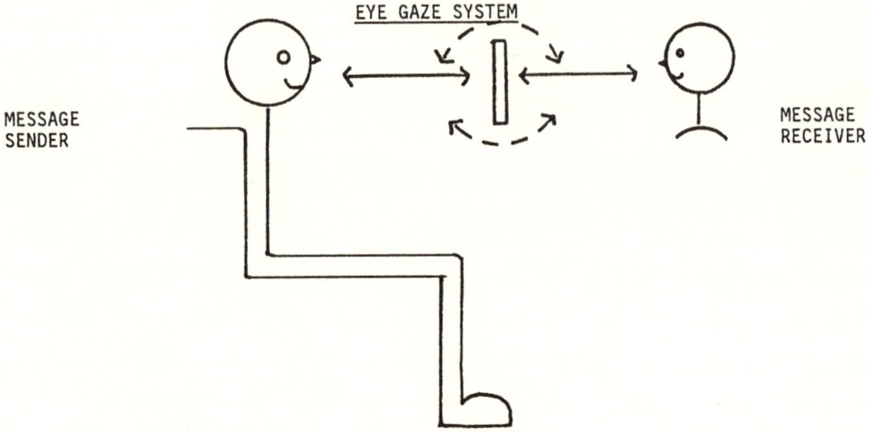

DISTANCE FROM USER'S FACE:______________________________

DISTANCE FROM SENDER'S FACE:______________________________

ANGLE:______________________________

MOUNTING OPTIONS:______________________________

____

____

____

ADDITIONAL COMMENTS:

RESOURCES:

Form C(1)

COMMUNICATION BOARD

NAME:____________ DATE:________ FAMILY ADVISOR:____________

DOB:________ NCMH #:________ COMMUNITY ADVOCATE:____________

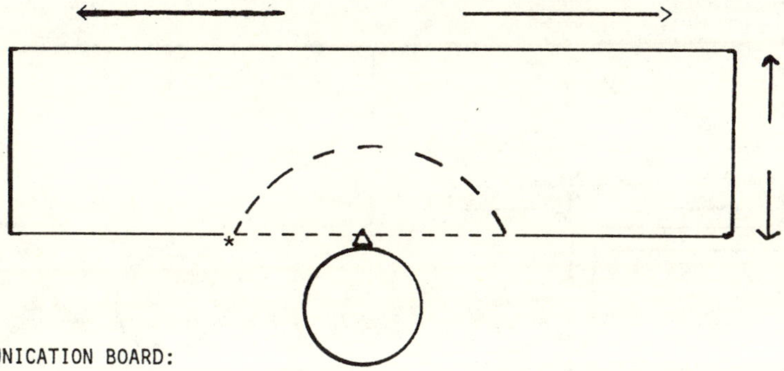

COMMUNICATION BOARD:

DIMENSIONS____________ *SIZE OF CUTOUT________

TYPE OF SYMBOLS TO BE DISPLAYED____________

SIZE OF LOCATION (SYMBOL SIZE)____________

DISTANCE BETWEEN SYMBOLS____________

NUMBER OF LOCATIONS TO BE DISPLAYED____________

FORMAT OF SYMBOLS____________

PLACEMENT OF SYMBOLS WITHIN RANGE OF INDICATION____________

____________ (RANGE AND DIMENSIONS OF RANGE ARE DRAWN ON THE GRAPHIC ABOVE)

EXAMPLE OF SYMBOL TO BE DISPLAYED:

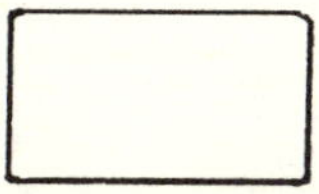

PLACEMENT/MOUNTING OPTIONS:

(1) Seated ____________

(2) Side Lying ____________

(3) Other ____________
(graphic of mounting on next page)

Form C(2)

ADDITIONAL COMMENTS:

RESOURCES:

COMMUNICATION BOARD SUMMARY

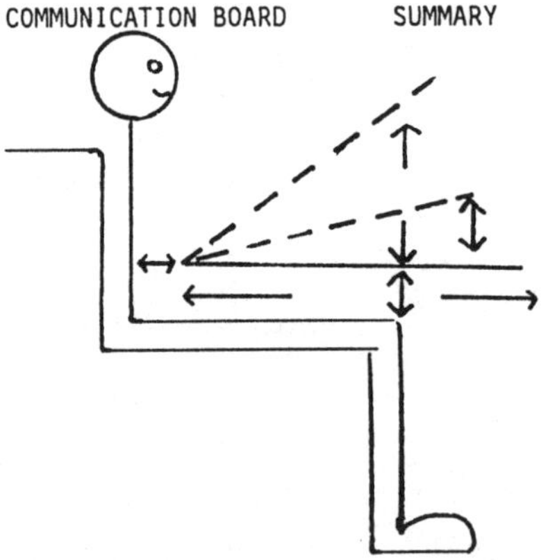

POSITIONING

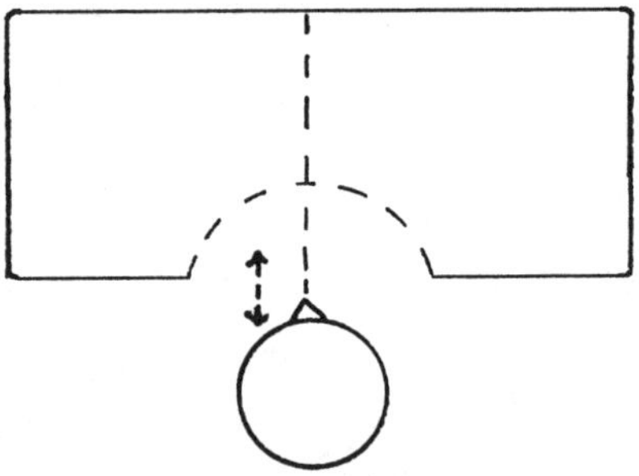

PLACEMENT

GRAPHIC OF MOUNTING OPTIONS:

SEATED

SIDE LYING

OTHER

Form D

COMMERCIAL DEVICE

NAME:____________________ DATE:_____________ FAMILY ADVISOR:_________________

DOB:___________ NCMH #____________ COMMUNITY ADVOCATE:______________________

DESCRIPTION OF DEVICE:____

____

INTERFACE:____

SYMBOL SYSTEM:____

RANGE OF INDICATION (with graphic):____

____

DISPLAY OPTIONS:____

____

____

MOUNTING OPTIONS (with graphic):____

____

____

ADDITIONAL COMMENTS:

RESOURCES:

APPENDIX II: RESOURCES ON COMMUNICATION AND COMPUTER TECHNOLOGY

This is a partial listing of resources. For a more extensive listing, see *The Exceptional Parent*, October, 1985.

INFORMATION CLEARINGHOUSES

American Speech-Language-Hearing Association (ASHA)
10801 Rockville Pike
Rockville, MD 20852

International Society for Augmentative and
Alternative Communication (ISAAC)
P.O. Box 1762
Station R
Toronto, Ontario M4G 4A3
Canada

Association for Special Education Technology
P.O. Box 152
Allen, TX 75002

Special Education Software Center
LINK Resources, Inc.
3857 N. High St.
Columbus, OH 43214

The Technical Resource Center
1820 Richmond Rd. SW
Calgary ALB T2T 5C7
Canada

Trace Research and Development Center
S. 151, 1500 Highland Ave.
Madison, Wisconsin 53706

PUBLICATIONS

Closing the Gap
P.O. Box 68
Henderson, MN 56044

Communication Outlook
Artificial Language Laboratory
Michigan State University
East Lansing, MI 48824

Computer Disability News
National Easter Seal Society
2023 W. Ogden Ave.
Chicago, IL 60612

COMMERCIAL VENDORS

Adaptive Communication Systems, Inc.
P.O. Box 12440
Pittsburgh, PA 15231

Adaptive Peripherals
4529 Bagley Ave. N.
Seattle, WA 98013

Apple Computer, Inc.
20525 Mariani Ave.
Cupertino, CA 95014

Artificial Language Laboratory
Michigan State University
East Lansing, MI 48824

Canon U.S.A., Inc.
One Canon Plaza
Lake Success, NY 11042-9979

Don Johnston Developmental Equipment
981 Winnetka Terr.
Lake Zurich, IL 60047

Handicapped Children's Technological Services
P.O. Box 7
Foster, RI 02825

Intex Micro Systems, Corp.
725 S. Adams Rd. Suite L8
Birmingham, MI 48011

J.A. Preston Corp.
60 Page Rd.
Clifton, NJ 07012

Laureate Learning Systems, Inc.
1 Mill St.
Burlington, VT 05401

Prentke Romich Co.
1022 Heyl Rd.
Wooster, OH 44691

Shea Products, Inc.
1042 W. Hamlin Rd.
Rochester, MI 48063

TASH, Inc.
70 Gibson Dr. Unit 1
Markham, Ontario L3R 2Z3
Canada

Texas Instruments
Software and Acquisition
P.O. Box 2909
Austin, TX 78769

Unicorn Engineering Co.
6201 Harwood Ave.
Oakland, CA 94618

Votan
4487 Technology Dr.
Freemont, CA 94538

Words +
1125 Stewert Ct. Suite D
Sunnyvale, CA 94086

Zygo Industries, Inc.
P.O. Box 1008
Portland, OR 92707